Leslie Blanchard's
Foolproof Guide to Beautiful Hair Color

Leslie Blanchard's
FOOLPROOF GUIDE TO BEAUTIFUL HAIR COLOR

Leslie Blanchard with Maureen Lynch

E. P. Dutton   New York

Published in the United States by E. P. Dutton,
a division of New American Library,
2 Park Avenue, New York, N.Y. 10016.

Library of Congress Cataloging-in-Publication Data
Blanchard, Leslie.
    Leslie Blanchard's foolproof guide to beautiful hair
color.
Includes index.
1. Hair—Dyeing and bleaching. 2. Beauty, Personal.
I. Lynch, Maureen. II. Title.
TT973.B54   1986   646.7'242   86-11441

ISBN:0-525-24457-3

Published simultaneously in Canada by
Fitzhenry & Whiteside Limited, Toronto

Designed by Jackie Schuman

10 9 8 7 6 5 4 3 2 1
First Edition

Hundreds of thousands of women have come to me over the years looking for help, advice, and inspiration, but there are sixteen women who are especially close to my heart. Each of them opened her life to me, was willing to be interviewed, to be photographed, and to share her personal story so other women might benefit from her experience. And so, with gratitude to them for inspiring me so deeply, I lovingly dedicate this book to the sixteen women whose stories and make-overs appear on the following pages.

[L.B.]

CONTENTS

Sixteen pages of color photographs follow page 88.

INTRODUCTION

I didn't pay much attention to the ringing telephone. The Elizabeth Arden salon in Fort Lauderdale, Florida, was very busy that winter season, with clients calling daily to have their hair done for the charity balls and parties that were scheduled each night. But when the manager hung up after one particular call, she whispered something to her assistant and suddenly everyone was whispering. I was putting the finishing touches on one of my clients when I noticed hurried sweeping-up, frantic clearing of counters, and the manager rushing down the aisle spraying Blue Grass cologne in the air. She stopped in front of me and said, "Mrs. Arden is on her way and you're going to do her hair, Leslie."

"Me? Mrs. Arden? You mean *the* Elizabeth Arden?" I sputtered. "What does she look like?"

"You'll find out soon enough," the manager shot back over her shoulder as she raced to the front door just as Mrs. Arden's chauffeur was handing the great lady out of her limousine.

I said a fast prayer and tried to swallow my fear as Elizabeth Arden herself was ushered into her salon and guided to my chair. She was a legend in the beauty business, the head of a gigantic empire, a regal woman with imperious bearing. And here she was, sitting in front of *me.* I was not only supposed to touch her hair, but make it look wonderful. I was twenty-two years old, looked fifteen, and it was one of the scariest moments of my young life.

Somehow I managed to calm down, draw a deep breath, and begin to comb her hair. Right away Mrs. Arden interrupted. "No, no, young man. You must first massage my Eight Hour Cream into my scalp before proceeding."

"Of course, Mrs. Arden," I responded. "I'd be delighted. I'm sorry I'm not familiar with your preferences, but I've been here just a short time. It's a great honor for me to have the opportunity to take care of you, and if you'll tell me a little more about how you like your hair done, I'm sure we can produce a result that will please you."

There was a long, *long* pause.

"All right, young man," she said finally. "You seem to know what you're about, so go ahead and do what you think is right."

Elizabeth Arden was my first famous client. At the time, she must have been in her seventies, but she still had wonderful posture and incredible "presence." And while she herself was not beautiful in the classic sense of the word, she was enormously sensitive to beauty and surrounded herself with it. She believed that beauty not only enhanced a person's life, but that it was an inalienable right, up there with life, liberty, and the pursuit of happiness. And she devoted her formidable energies to the belief that you must *care deeply* about beauty in order to produce it.

In many ways, Mrs. Arden sowed the seeds of what became my own professional creed: Every woman in the world is beautiful. All she has to do is to get in touch with that beauty. Mrs. Arden was a great inspiration, and although she was my very first famous client, she certainly wasn't my last. Since then, I've worked with almost every film, stage, television, or society personality you'd like to name. But I'm getting ahead of myself. First, let me tell you a little about my background and how I started in this wonderful business.

I'm a small-town boy, born in East Barre, Vermont, population six hundred and located smack in the middle of the state. It's a beautiful part of the country and when the leaves start turning in the fall, people drive hundreds of miles to admire nature's spectacular display. My mother worked part time as the village postmistress and my father was district sales manager for a local granite manufacturer. There were five of us, my parents, my brother, and my grandmother, who had been widowed and moved into the other half of our two-family house when I was still quite young. I was the eldest grandchild and loved the extra attention I received from "Gram." When I'd come home from school, she'd be there with milk and cookies and we'd talk about all sorts of things. She taught me how to garden and how to plant flower beds according to color families that looked harmonious together. She taught me to cook, too, since she'd be starting the evening meal while my mother was still at work. Each person in our family, and in our town, for that matter, did what he or she did best to contribute to our lives together. And everyone really cared for everyone else, with a sense of giving and sharing I feel I've been able to carry into my adult life and profession.

Although my early years were happy times, I was always a restless child. One night when we were listening to Lux Radio Theatre, I picked up a hairbrush lying nearby and began to brush Gram's hair. It was fun and she seemed to like it. So each night we'd sit together listening to the radio while I brushed her hair. A few weeks later, when we came in from a gardening session, I helped her shampoo her hair at the kitchen sink. Then she showed me how to set her hair. I enjoyed that, too. Most of all, I loved the way she looked with her hair freshly shampooed and set. She was very pretty in my young eyes.

Besides being restless, I seemed to have lots of energy. By age twelve I was delivering newspapers in our village and by fourteen I was helping out in our country store every day after school and over holiday vacations. By then I had started to take some business courses in high school and was eager to apply those lessons to real-life situations. The post office was right next to the store so my mother was able not only to keep an eye on me but to guide and teach me in those first work days. Standing behind the counter in that country store in a small town in Vermont, I learned how to listen to my customers—to what they wanted or needed and what would make them happy. It was an experience that has stayed with me through my entire professional life.

Music was part of my education, too. I was pretty good on the violin and played in the school orchestra. When we played for the basketball team, though, I switched to the French horn. I'd learned how to play it because it meant I could travel with the band when we played for the team's "away" games. It was on one of those school trips to Boston that my future was determined.

My family knew a woman from Barre who had married a man who owned a beauty school in Boston. They arranged for me to meet Mr. and Mrs. Behns. Between band practices, I went to see them and the Wilfred Beauty School. I felt at home immediately. I remember to this day having a sense of belonging there, so I made a decision on the spot that after high school graduation, that's where I would go. I was only sixteen years old at the time, but I was so comfortable with that decision that I never wavered from it or questioned it again. It felt right and that was that.

Had it not been for the French horn and the basketball team's schedule, I might have been a floral designer or a chef, since I've never lost my passions for food and flowers. But fate had decreed beauty school and that was what I was going to do.

As soon as I finished high school, I entered Wilfred's and learned all the traditional hairdressing skills. It turned out to be a very good choice for me. I was hired immediately by a salon in Boston, where I worked for the next three years. Many of my clients were young college girls with a great sense of adventure who loved experimenting with their hair. And I loved being their accomplice. Besides trying different styles, we had great fun playing with different hair-color effects. The results were always dramatic: either perfectly fabulous or totally disastrous! When I look back on what we tried . . . and with absolutely *no* fear of the consequences! But we all had great fun and learned in the process. I discovered I loved working with color more than anything, even though hair color at that time (in the mid 1950s) had no subtlety to it at all. Blondes were either brassy yellow or white. Reds were orange or pink. And all the browns looked like chocolate pudding. I loved hair coloring anyhow. Cuts and styles could come and go, but I realized the color of the hair was the "fabric" of hair design. Just as a good fashion designer starts with the most beautiful material, I started to invent my own color formulas that would show off the richness and texture of the hair. I didn't realize at the time that I'd found my professional specialty.

Next came that fateful winter in Florida at the Elizabeth Arden salon that I've already told you about. As the end of that season approached, a woman from Saks Fifth Avenue asked me if I would come to New York with her for some additional training, then travel around the country to teach other stylists how to color hair. That woman's name was Iris Segal and she worked for the company that leased hundreds of beauty salons in department stores (including Saks).

I thought it sounded like a great idea and so, at age twenty-three, I became a teacher and trainer of stylists, specializing in hair color technique. It was Mrs. Segal who told me, "Leslie, you will be very famous, but it will take a long time because what you do with hair color is so subtle. Also, many women won't want to admit they color their hair."

She was right on all counts. My formulas were so new that most people didn't know what to make of them. And there was still some social censure attached to coloring your hair. Nonetheless, my work continued to flourish and after traveling for about a year, I was called back to New York to do nothing but teach. My new responsibilities took just a few hours of my time each evening and because I was (and am) very energetic, I started going into the Saks salon for a few hours every day to help my clients with any color problems they were having. It was something I loved doing, working with both the clients and the stylists.

At this same time, word reached Clairol, this country's major manufacturer of hair-coloring products, that there was a "new kid on the block" over at Saks who really seemed to know what he was doing. They approached me about becoming a consultant to help them with new product development and publicity as well as to lead seminars and training sessions. I agreed, and it was the beginning of a twenty-year relationship. Working as Clairol's chief color consultant was a very satisfying part of my career.

While with Clairol, though, I did make one huge mistake. I was scheduled to appear in a commercial for a new coloring product. I wasn't used to being in *front* of the camera . . . usually I was *behind* the camera putting the last touches on the model's hair. But there I was, slated for stardom, or so they said. Since I had already begun to go bald, I let myself be convinced that I should be fitted for a hairpiece. I was nervous and wasn't thinking straight. I did the commercial while wearing the hairpiece, which I *hated*, and I looked and sounded on camera just the way I felt, stiff and artificial. But that experience taught me a great lesson, one that I still pass on to my clients every day: If you try to look too different and go too far from your normal appearance, you'll never come across in a natural way. I know that for a fact, having tried it myself!

At the same time that I was teaching and working with Clairol, Saks Fifth Avenue set up a special salon for me, called the Leslie Blanchard Color Studio. We were overwhelmed with bookings, because not only was there a great demand for good hair color, we were one of the few (if *only*) places to go that *specialized* in color. Besides our regular clients, we did all the stars—Inger Stevens, Carroll Baker, Paulette Goddard, Gloria Swanson. There wasn't a major film or Broadway star who didn't check in with us.

Joan Fontaine was one of them. Since finishing *Tender Is the Night* she'd moved from California to New York and had let her hair go back to its natural color, which was *not* very colorful. She has fine, fragile hair and wasn't sure what to do with it. I told her, "With your beautiful skin and bone structure, your hair should be simple and elegant, so everyone can really see who you are. A soft golden-blonde shade would be perfect for you. I'd like to see you in a smooth, simple style with the hair worn back off your face." That's just what we did for her and she's worn her hair in variations of that theme ever since.

I consider the 1960s the time when modern hair color really took off and started to become the boon to beauty we know today. Formulations were developed that were more gentle to the hair and the number of shades from which you could choose multiplied like crazy. Although this was the decade of protest and hippies, the Leslie Blanchard Color Studio at Saks Fifth Avenue continued to do a booming business with women who wanted their hair to look its best, even if they *were* wearing jeans. In fact, business was so good and I developed such a following of clients, that in 1970 I drew a very deep breath and opened my own salon on the second floor of a building in the East Sixties of Manhattan between Fifth and Madison avenues. I called it the Private World of Leslie Blanchard, because I wanted women to feel at home there, to feel comfortable and confident that we would be taking the best care of them and their hair. In 1975 we expanded to two other floors, and in 1979 I bought the whole building.

Most days, that's where you'll find me, giving consultations and working with my clients. I'm there because I love being there. I feel very blessed to have chosen a career that is filled with such satisfaction. I love going to work every day because, by the evening, I know I will have helped several women achieve their utmost beauty potential and showed them a new, beautiful way to feel good about themselves. I guess my enthusiasm shows, because in the last couple of years, I've been asked to do hundreds of guest appearances on television—"Good Morning America," "Today," "The Morning Show," "A.M. Los Angeles," "America," and "The Oprah Winfrey Show" in Chicago. Oprah said to me recently, "Leslie, you always seem so happy and willing to give away all your good advice. Do you really feel that way?"

"I love it," I told her. "I want every woman in this country to look magical and marvelous. The more advice I give away, the better women will look, and the better they look, the more time I'll have to have fun in my kitchen and garden."

These television appearances have taken my career in a direction I never could have predicted, and I must admit I love the immediacy of the medium. What's more, I love getting out of my salon into smaller cities and towns when I do shows on the road. I meet women there that I'd never get to meet in New York. It's exciting, educational, and informative for me, just as the women I do on television say it is for them. But as much fun as television make-overs can be, they don't give me much time to explain to each woman I meet what she can do with her own hair color at home.

Traveling around the country as I do, I've come to realize that for every woman I see in my salon or during a television make-over, there are hundreds and possibly thousands more I could be helping with solid professional guidance. That is my most important reason for taking the time to write this book. I want to give you all the encouragement, information, and assurance I can that you really can do your hair color yourself and do it *well.*

There is nothing mysterious about coloring your hair, and yet, I know, it can seem a very scary prospect. Remember the first time you tried an ambitious recipe in the kitchen? It may have looked difficult, but once you did it, you saw how easy it really was. Hair coloring is like that. Changing your image can be daunting, too. You may not be happy with the way you look now, but at least you know what you're dealing with. Changing all that can feel like stepping off the edge of a cliff. You may be saying to yourself, What if it doesn't look right when I'm finished? How do I pick the right color? Will I be making things worse?

Trust me. I really know what I'm talking about and have spent the last thirty years of my professional life not only developing the data bank of information on hair color, but learning the tips and tricks of the trade that only day-after-day experience can teach. And you're about to get every single bit of that inside information. It's possible that I may know more about hair color than any other single individual in the world. Don't forget that I've been coloring hair all this time, plus I've had extensive experience on the technical side, too, developing new products and ways to use them best.

And in case you're still nervous, remember I've been *teaching* hair color to hairstylists for many years, and believe me, if I can teach other professionals, I promise I can teach you, too. After all, I consider you a professional in your own right. Who knows your face and hair better than you do? And you've learned to use makeup like a pro, haven't you? With a little guidance, you'll be able to do your own hair color, too.

Besides being anxious about taking the plunge and coloring your hair, you may feel some trepidation about the commitment of "keeping it up" afterward. Let me tell you something amazing. In all the years I've been coloring hair and hearing from the hundreds of thousands of women whose hair I've done, I have yet to hear a *single* woman come back to complain that the commitment wasn't worth the effort! Once you start being deluged with compliments and have been told over and over again how great you look, you'll *want* to keep it up. Spending a small amount of time caring for yourself to keep your looks in tip-top shape will become a *joy.* You don't mind caring for loved ones, do you? Taking a little care of yourself will give you the same sense of satisfaction.

Well, now it's time to begin. By the time you finish reading this book you'll know all you need to know about handling your hair color comfortably and with confidence. I want you to succeed in this. I really, truly *care* about you. I want you to be the most beautiful woman you can be. I want you to look and feel perfectly wonderful. So come on, we'll do this together. Put your hand in mine, and let's get started.

Part One

INSPIRATION

1
How Changing Your Hair Can Change Your Life

What does your hair look like right now? Is it dull, drab, too brassy, or a "no color" mixture of gray and brown? Have you been thinking about "doing something" with your hair? If you have determined there's room for improvement, you've already taken the first step toward maximizing your good looks. Your hair probably *would* look better if it were brighter, livelier, more colorful, and, consequently, more flattering. And if you've been thinking about making a change, you've come to the right place.

Over the years, thousands of women have asked me to "do something" with their hair. In every single case, the woman has experienced a growing suspicion that her hair could look a lot better. Each has realized in her own way that the better she looks, the better she is going to feel about herself. Each is looking for the wonderful "lift" great-looking hair offers. To me, that's what looking your best is all about. It makes you feel terrific inside.

Can simply changing your hair accomplish that? You bet it can! Short of losing a substantial amount of weight, changing your hair is the single most dramatic improvement you can make in your looks. I've seen it happen over and over again. Women come into my salon looking timid, unsure, and tentative. They leave standing tall, smiling, radiating confidence and self-esteem. Being able to enhance a woman's sense of herself and being able to see the results so dramatically is what I love best about what I do and what has kept me doing it for over thirty years. I know how wonderful you can feel when you know you look terrific, and I want to encourage you in any way I can to draw a deep breath and take the plunge.

Dramatic versus Radical Change

In describing a hair change as dramatic I do not necessarily mean a radical change. A dramatic effect can be achieved with very little. It could be as simple as adding some discreet highlights. That change, however, brings your face and hair into a harmony that wasn't present before and, in that sense, produces a dramatic effect. The same would hold true for a woman who has just enough gray to obscure her hair color. Covering the gray or using it to highlight her face in a flattering way is another change that is *not* radical but does have a dramatic effect.

In deciding how much change to make in a woman's looks, I tend to think like a conservative plastic surgeon. I don't want you to look so different you feel you have to give explanations to friends or family. But I do want you to look wonderful, with a new sparkle. If your friends can't quite put their finger on why you look especially pretty, that's perfect! They may say, "You've done something to your hair" or "You've changed your makeup." What they mean is, "You look terrific." And while changing your hair isn't nearly as permanent as cosmetic surgery, I don't want whatever change you make to be so profound that you feel you've lost touch with the person you see in the mirror.

How Much Change Can You Handle?

If you were to come to me in person, before I looked closely at your hair I would ask you some key questions about yourself and your life. Do you consider yourself an introvert or an extravert? Or are you, like most of us, somewhere in the middle? Do you like to be "in charge" most of the time or are you more comfortable "going with the flow"? Are you constantly meeting new people or do you live in a fairly stable community? How many black-tie dinner dances did you attend in the last year? How many times did you stand up to speak in front of a group in the last six months? On a daily basis, how many hours do you spend in your car? Your office? Your home? And, most important, how much time are you willing to spend on hair care? Daily? Monthly?

Of course, if we were talking in person, you and I would get into a full discussion at this point. Nonetheless, these preliminary questions are good ones to ask yourself on your own, right now. They will help you focus on how much of a statement you want your hair to make about you and will help you determine how much change you can comfortably handle. And since the chapters in Part Two of this book are arranged according to the degree of change each coloring method will have on your hair's appearance, starting with temporary color (the least amount of change) on through allover frosting (the most dramatic change), you'll begin to develop a very good idea of which coloring method would suit you best.

You may be ready for substantial change. Recently a schoolteacher came to me for help. She wanted a "total make-over." Prematurely gray since college days, she'd begun to suspect that, decades later, her gray hair was too aging for her. Looking at her college reunion photos really convinced her. She said, "I felt I looked like everyone else's mother." To me, her hair appeared black and white and not at all flattering. After trimming her hair into a more contemporary style, I colored her hair a soft brown with taupe highlights. The next day, her husband of thirty years sent her roses. The next week, she found her students were much more attentive. Shedding her "grandmother" image was an enormous change for that woman, but one she wanted and one she's delighted she made.

All you need may be a small, but significant, change. Actress Kathleen Turner found herself in that situation. Because she'd been working continuously and ignoring her hair, her natural blonde had begun to look drab and colorless. I decided she needed just a scattering of blonde highlights to brighten her looks. That's what I started to give her, but then she was cast as the female lead in *Prizzi's Honor* opposite Jack Nicholson, which required she be a very glamorous blonde. For her movie role, I lightened her hair just that way. But once the movie was shot and she was back in private life, sunny highlights were all she needed to complement her natural beauty. This is a good example of a small change that makes a big difference.

Keeping Up with Your Life

Besides, How much change can I handle?, a good question to ask yourself is, Does my hair go with the rest of my life? You may find that the decisions you made about your hair several years ago don't work as well as they used to. This happens very frequently.

When Barbara Walters first left her writer's desk on the "Today" show to go in front of the camera, her hair was so dark it looked dense black on-screen. Initially, I lightened her hair to a warm brown that photographed better and made her look prettier without looking any less in command. Over a period of twenty years, I've gradually lightened her hair so it is now a very light brown with golden highlights. In my view, Barbara Walters has never looked better. She's at the acme of her career and looks just like what she is—a glamorous professional.

Classic beauty Alexis Smith is another woman who has kept her looks in step with her life. She's always had reddish-blonde hair, but has constantly shifted its emphasis to suit her activities. For her Broadway role in *Follies,* I brightened her hair to dramatize her impact onstage and underscore her "star" image.

While you may not have to update your looks continuously to suit stage lights or a camera, you can still draw a very valuable lesson from women who lead their lives in the public eye: They regularly adjust their looks to suit the way they are living their lives *that minute!* No "waiting until . . ." for them. For *you*, being aware of emphasis changes in your own life will truly help you to keep your looks in top form.

Right now I'm thinking of two of my private clients, both of whom are the same age, thirty-nine. One has just seen her eldest child off to college. The other has quit a high-powered job to stay home with her new baby. The college mom now has a little more time to spend on herself and is looking for more sophistication in her hairstyle. The new mother needs super-easy-care hair. Both are making changes that are compatible with the way their lives are evolving *at this time.*

Milestone Make-overs

In the pages that follow, you are going to see lots of examples of women who made a decision to change their looks and who enhanced their lives in the process. Although women have many more options today than ever before (you do not have to be married by age twenty-two, have a career on track by thirty, and stop having children at thirty-five), there are still certain important milestones that most women use as turning points, moments at which they pause to take stock of their lives. With those in mind, we've organized our Before-and-After make-overs along the lines of these classic milestones.

My hope is that you will see yourself in one or more of our stories and realize that you, too, can change your looks for the better. Further, I've cross-referenced each of our women according to the hair-coloring method I used to enhance her looks. In each case, I will give you a complete explanation of what I did and how you can duplicate the look yourself, at home, on your own. In the second part of this book, starting with chapter 7, How to Color Your Hair at Home, I will share with you all the tips and tricks I've developed in my thirty years as a professional. I'm glad to share my expertise with you, because it is my fervent wish that you be able to benefit from my experience. I want you to have that soul-satisfying feeling that you've never looked better or felt so good about yourself in your whole life.

Now, on with our stories.

2

Starting Out

I hear that comment all the time from young women in their twenties. The first few years after school are when most young women begin to set directions for their lives, starting a career, marrying, having a baby, continuing their education, or all of the above. For many, these are the years devoted to establishing who they are and who they are going to be in the future. It's a wonderful and exciting time in a woman's life. To see an individual at this age is to see her in her first full flowering as a woman. No longer a "girl," she has just begun to have a glowing sense of pride and confidence in herself.

Sometimes, however, a young woman's looks may not be projecting the way she feels about herself inside. Her looks may have to be adjusted, refocused, reestablished if that young woman is to feel comfortable with herself and what's she's doing with her life.

The single most important thing this young woman must do if she wants to be perceived as an adult is to get rid of the hairstyle she had in high school or college. Nothing can freeze-frame a young woman faster than looking the same way she did in her yearbook photo. If you look in the mirror today and see the same image you had senior year, it's time for a change. So much has happened in your life over the last few years that you *owe* it to yourself to keep your looks moving forward, too! If you want to be taken seriously, you have to look as if your take *yourself* seriously!

If you've already accepted the responsibilities of an adult, don't you want to look that way, too? Wouldn't it be better for you to look like a competent young mother than a cheerleader? How about your career? Don't you think you'll be promoted faster if you assume the image of a professional instead of cruising along in your high school hairdo? I don't mean to suggest that the suspicion your looks may be on overtime hasn't already occurred to you. It probably has. What I'm encouraging you to do is to take some action, this minute, to bring your looks into harmony with your new adult status in life.

You remember the years of carefree play you experienced as a child, summers at the beach, the lake, playing outdoors in the field. The sun probably brightened your hair at the time, making it look beautiful and vibrant. But now that you're no longer a child and are living in the grown-up world, you may feel your looks have dimmed a bit in the last few years. Perhaps your skin tone or eyes don't look as bright as you think they once did. It may be time for you to turn the lights back on, to enhance your best features, to glorify your hair and reestablish some excitement in your looks.

I'm not implying you should try to turn the clock back to look like a child again. That's going in reverse. Instead, I want you to step on the accelerator and start using what you have naturally to look your super best. I want you to develop an attitude of confidence, of being beautiful inside and out. I want you to enjoy the burgeoning sense of security you have in yourself.

If what I'm saying here strikes a chord with you, let me take you a few steps further by introducing you to four young women who feel the way you do about yourself and who have gone ahead to change their looks in exciting ways.

Jan Kennedy

Age 28
Fullerton, California
Wife, mother, actress
"I have a new, more exciting
view of myself."

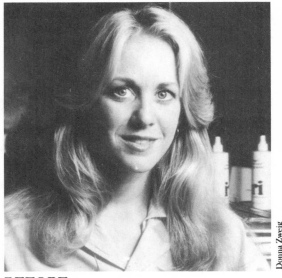

BEFORE

"My hair still looks like it did in high school," Jan wrote in her letter to me. "It's naturally blonde, bone straight, and reaches the middle of my back. I think I'm ready for a change."

The picture she attached to her note showed Jan with her two beautiful children, ages five and two. Her description of herself was totally accurate: She still looked like a teenager. I was in Los Angeles at the time, looking for make-over candidates for the "A.M. Los Angeles" television show. I felt Jan would be perfect for the program. She was the ideal California blonde, leggy, tall, outdoorsy, with a wonderful figure and all that fabulous hair, yet she was really itching for a change.

When we met, Jan told me more about herself. She'd been a cheerleader in high school as well as vice-president of the student council, editor of the annual, and homecoming princess. She'd married her high school sweetheart, whom she'd dated since she was fifteen, and now lived near her parents. While her family life was a source of great satisfaction and stability to Jan, she was feeling restless about herself and her looks. "I'm ready to begin my life as an adult," is the way she described herself.

"What really did it," she added, "was having my tenth high school reunion and my tenth wedding anniversary the same month. When I looked at the pictures taken at both events, I realized that, except for a little normal aging, I still looked very much the same. Yet so much had happened to me in those ten years since school! I felt that in one way the time had flown by, but my appearance had stayed put and made me look like I was still a kid. I really want to look as if I'm grown up now."

Jan's instinct was right. She isn't a cheerleader anymore. She has other needs, other goals, other achievements in her life. She's a young woman who has taken on the responsibilities of an adult and she *deserves* to look the part she's earned for herself. She's a wife, a mother of two young children, is going to acting classes full time, and has already had a few small parts in films and television movies. Her life has simply outdistanced her high school looks.

Jan's hair has always been a fabulous asset, but when I first met her, it was dragging her down. It was too long, too heavy, and the natural blonde color had dulled just enough to dim the light in her beautiful skin. Her hair desperately needed to be freed up so that her natural energy and bounce could come through. And she needed a much more exciting style to give her versatility beyond that monotonous, straight-haired look, both for her private life and for her professional objectives.

Looking at Jan's face, I noticed that her complexion was beginning to show early signs of overexposure, a result of spending a lot of time outdoors. Although Jan protects her skin, I felt she needed even more protection—and a little more makeup! On first impression, no one feature of Jan's stood out, they all ran together with none of them pointed up

or highlighted. I knew that if I didn't see any definition in Jan's face, neither would anyone else. And yet Jan has *gorgeous* blue eyes. I wanted to create more personality for her, to define her looks more, to bring out those sparkling blue eyes, and to give her more glamour! Here was a young woman with all the potential in the world to look devastatingly beautiful and exciting!

Jan's fabulous hair looks as if it's been released from prison. It's free, loose, dramatic, glamorous, and sophisticated. Hair like Jan's will always command attention. There is no way she can ever sneak quietly into a room and not be noticed. That's why her hair should *always* look bright, glorious, and be shown off to its fullest potential as Jan's "crowning glory."

"I absolutely *love* it," she told me as we finished. "There's a wildness to it that I just *adore* instead of that same old boring hairdo."

Jan had everything she needed to dramatize her looks. We started by controlling the volume of her hair with a graduated cut that broke up the dense thickness and gave her hair an open, airy feeling. I wanted to see color that looked as if soft sunlight were streaming through her hair, so we added some sparkling highlights to emphasize her golden, California-blonde good looks. The color we then washed through Jan's hair not only added more glow and a feeling of sunshine in her hair, it also brought out those wonderful blue eyes (see chapter 14, Frosting).

Jan loves colors and has the looks, energy, and excitement to wear them beautifully. That's why she can go as far as she likes with her makeup, using two or three different colors of eye shadow and a bold, clear lipstick. She can wear the most colorful fashion, too, since her hair has already set her image in a dramatic direction. Jan has the world by the tail now and she has every reason to swing it!

"I have such a wonderful new feeling about myself," she told me. "I'm much more confident walking into an audition. And my husband loves the way I look, too. We finished my make-over just in time for New Year's Eve. He bought me a fabulous new dress for the occasion, so all our friends could see the 'new me.' But there's more to it than just my new looks. I really feel like a grown-up now . . . inside *and* out."

Jan had been ready for a change. I'm thrilled that dramatizing her natural good looks helped put her in touch with herself again and gave her the feeling that new doors were opening for her in all areas of her life.

Jan's makeup, and the makeup of all the women in this book, was done by makeup artist Louis Bonadio.

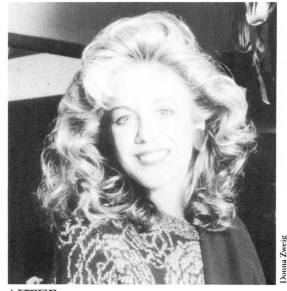

AFTER

Donna Zweig

Karen Risi

Age 29
Jackson Heights, New York
Import expediter
"A polished image counts in my business."

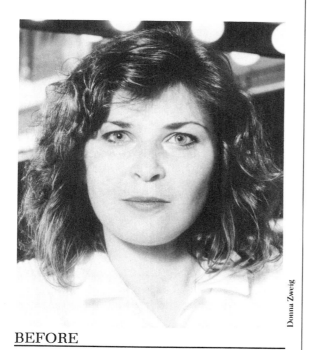

Donna Zweig

BEFORE

Karen came to me as a client the same way many women do, when they hear from friends that I really care about the way they look and want to help them look their best. Karen was aware of my reputation, then checked further with some model friends to be sure she was going to the right person. The reason she was particularly cautious was that she'd had a bad perm four years before and didn't want to repeat a negative experience. She simply didn't want to gamble again. As she said in our consultation, "It took over a year and a half for that bad perm to grow out and all during that time I felt I wanted to hide under the covers. But you can't bury your hair in a drawer and forget it like a sweater you don't want to wear anymore."

I understood Karen's caution. Since I never saw the problematic perm, however, there was no way for me to evaluate where the choices of cut or perm had gone wrong on her particular hair. I could see what had happened since, though. Because Karen didn't know quite what to do with her looks, she'd done nothing. When I looked at her, the first thing I saw were these incredible gray-green eyes. It was like looking into a deep green sea. Talk about sensational! But with the way her hair was styled, or *un*styled, the hair was falling across her forehead and casting a shadow over her eyes.

And although Karen's skin is very fair, it seemed to have very little light or glow to it, probably because the color of her dark hair was so nondescript. Also,

Karen's face is fullest at the cheeks and her dark hair was accentuating their fullness by creating too much of a contrast at that part of her face.

As we talked, I discovered Karen thought of herself as a blonde! That's what she put on her driver's license. You may find that difficult to believe, looking at her Before picture—and so did her husband, who kept saying to her, "Karen, you're *not* a blonde, you have brown hair." But in her heart of hearts, Karen was still a blonde, because that's the way she looked as a teenager spending summers in the sun. Once she started working full time in an office with no summer sun to lighten her hair, it darkened over a relatively short period of time.

Karen's looks needed refocusing and reestablishing because they were not in tune with her life or her career. She has lovely skin, those incredibly beautiful eyes, and was determined to get out of the beauty rut she'd fallen into. I thought she could look much, much prettier and more authoritative because that's the way she felt about herself.

Karen's blonde again, with a softer, smoother, more glamorous look than she ever had as a teenager. This time it's a blonde shade that suits an exciting, capable young woman. Karen works as an import expediter for a retail chain in the fashion field and she needed to look more a part of the business she's in. "I love projecting this image," she com-mented. "In my business, the way you look really counts. Everyone I work with is doing *something* to help her looks along and make the best of what she's got. And it's not only that. Now I look in the mirror and see Karen Risi, blonde."

To my eye, Karen's looks needed to be softened and integrated to create an impression of strong but quiet drama. We started by coloring her hair in a soft, cool blonde to maximize the impact of those incredible gray-green eyes. Color on Karen must be subtle. If she's *too* blonde or wears colors that are too sharp, they will disturb the delicate and beautiful balance of her fair skin and light eyes. We added a few extra highlights across the top of her hair to lighten her eyes even more, but did very few around the sides of her face, lest highlights in that area make her cheeks look even fuller (Chapter 11, Highlighting, especially comments on "cool" highlights). In that way, we used color to *contour* Karen's face the way a portrait painter would, not just to lighten her hair.

The sculpted, blunt cut we gave Karen added sleekness and polish to her looks. For her, a hairstyle must look as if it's been deliberately designed, not as if it happened by chance. With this type of cut, plus her soft, glowing color, the hair looks fuller and takes on gloss, shine, and drama. This is the way a young woman in Karen's business *should* look: chic and authoritative. Shape and line are very important in this style, as you see in the sweeping side bangs. It's a finished look that works perfectly for Karen.

The biggest challenge with Karen's makeup is not to interfere with the gorgeous color of her eyes or to overwhelm her face with color that would be too bright for her. That's why the eye shadow we used is muted and blended very thoroughly. We used a deep taupey gray color to add a little mystery and really bring out Karen's natural eye color. If you are lucky enough to have eyes this shade, whatever you do, avoid any shadow that is blue or yellow, or you will kill your wonderful color with incompatible makeup. Karen's eyeliner is gray-green to enhance her eyes, but it is drawn on with great economy, again, to complement, rather than compete with, the limpid beauty of her eyes. Anything heavier or darker would be a distraction. Her lipstick was kept in a soft, muted shade so as not to direct too much attention to the fullest part of her face. And blusher is on the quiet side, too, just a dusting of it over the cheeks to add a hint of color and highlight Karen's understated, fresh beauty.

When Karen went back to work after her make-over, she experienced a wonderful reaction from her colleagues. "My supervisor was very impressed," she told me. "Some people took a while to notice how different I looked, but all of them loved it. I guess I learned a big lesson," she continued. "You can't neglect your image. Looking the way I do now shows that I take myself more seriously, that I'm not frivolous. I'm very, very happy with what you did, Leslie. I feel I have a new way of looking at myself and

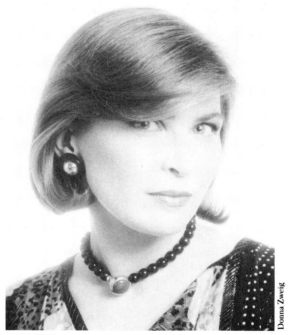

AFTER

Donna Zweig

I'm very, very comfortable with it."

A month after we worked together Karen received some wonderful news: She's pregnant. Since then, Karen has maintained her new image: "I wanted to keep up with the way my body was changing," she said. She's due to go on maternity leave next week and by the time you read this, she will have had her first baby, a joyful, happy, and blessed event for a lovely young woman.

Stephanie Tucker

Age 25
Seattle, Washington
Model/actress
"Sophistication suits me fine. . . .
I love it."

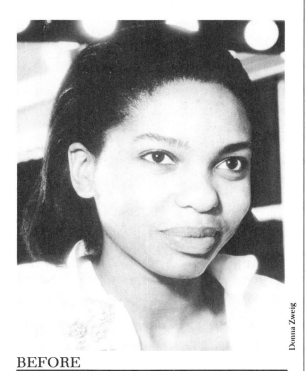

BEFORE

Donna Zweig

As an only child, Stephanie learned to rely on herself when she was very young, and at twenty-five is used to doing things on her own. That sense of independence has served her well in her professional life: She commutes between Seattle and New York, where she is both a photographic and free-lance runway model, specializing in bathing suits and sportswear. She maintains a rigorous schedule that gives her very little "down" time, and although she has to look *perfect* for work, she has very few hours to devote to her looks.

When we met, she told me, "I know something is just 'off' but I don't know what it is. I have so much hair, I sometimes tie it back in a ponytail just to get it out of the way. And it usually takes me six or seven hours to have it done in a salon because there's so much of it. I hate having to spend that much time on my hair. That's why I don't have it done as often as I should. I don't know if there's something else I can be doing, but I thought I'd at least ask you for any suggestions you might have."

I had plenty of suggestions. Stephanie is a beautiful brownette, but the glow was missing. Her hair looked dense and dark with no warmth or light filtering through it. Because of all the darkness in the hair, her eyes looked heavy and dense, too. Even her skin was being robbed of its vitality and was looking sallow, which in turn made her look just plain tired. Her hair was so thick, it overpowered her face, and, in the full-length view, made her look top-heavy, which was a shame, considering her stunning figure. She had "relaxed" her hair to make it more manageable, but in doing so, had dried it out. It was looking dull, flat, and nondescript. And all that thickness had the effect of making her face look rounder than it really is. We weren't seeing her great cheekbones, which are one of her best features.

When Stephanie tied her hair back, I got a really good look at her eyes, which are not only beautifully shaped, but contain light flecks of amber, adding a warm and fabulous dimension to her beauty. I wanted her to look more dynamic and dramatic, a look that would better match the feeling she has about herself inside—pride and sense of accomplishment.

There was a richness in Stephanie's looks begging to be brought out. We warmed up her hair so it would have gloss, shine, and reflect light, creating more of a glow. I explained to Stephanie that the reason I wanted to lighten her hair just a little is that it would make all the difference in how much light would suffuse not only her hair, but her face and eyes as well. The dark, dense hair had made her appear as if she were standing under a gray cloud. I knew she would be glorious with a bright, sunny look. The effect was like turning a light switch from Off to On. Although Stephanie is still (and should always be) a brownette, her hair color now has a softness and vibrancy to it that aims light at her beautiful face and

brings her looks into a new, dynamic harmony.

I first combed some highlights through Stephanie's hair to give it an extra bit of sunniness. We concentrated those highlights across the top to give her face a little more length. Then we washed a golden-brown color through her hair to give it an extra color lift (see chapter 14, Frosting). Stephanie told me that auburn hair runs in her family and it's in her hair, too. You can see a touch of it in her highlights.

While we cut her hair a little shorter on top to take away that heavy, flat look and permit her hair to have its natural, springy body, we didn't layer it at all. We didn't want to cut into any of her natural fullness that is a dream for any stylist to work with. Instead, we simply graduated her cut, making it shorter on top and wider at the sides to show off those cheekbones. We tapered the cut at the bottom so her neck would look longer and more regal. The shape of this cut is not only flattering to Stephanie, it is very versatile and permits her to change it around for her different modeling jobs.

With more light shining on her face, we could really go to town with Stephanie's new makeup. She wears all the pinks, lavenders, and purples beautifully and can take a lot of color well. But we blended and blended. There's a little iridescence in her eye shadow, but not too much to confuse her natural eye color. As you can see, the eye makeup took the heavy look away from Stephanie's eyes and made them look lighter. Even the whites of her eyes look brighter.

When we finished, Stephanie was *thrilled* with the way she looked. "I feel like an Egyptian queen," she told me. "It's such a relief to get out from under that mass of hair. I used to feel that my clients would see my hair first, then me. Now I feel I can walk into a studio and not have the hairstylist groan when he sees my hair. It's a much more professional look for me and I know it will look good under the lights."

There is nothing *plain* about Stephanie. She has a strong personality by nature and presents herself well every time she goes on an interview. I knew that with her radiant new looks, she'd be even more confident of herself.

A few weeks later Stephanie stopped by to tell me that her hair color and new makeup was making a big difference in her bookings. She was getting a lot more work. One long-time client asked, "Stephanie, are your eyes getting lighter? They really look different." But most of her clients couldn't pinpoint what she'd done to herself. They just knew she looked better than ever. The simple hair color change from a dark, dense brown to a lighter, warmer brown made a wonderful difference in Stephanie's looks and life. Her new hair plus dramatic new makeup gave a tremendous boost to Stephanie's natural sophistication.

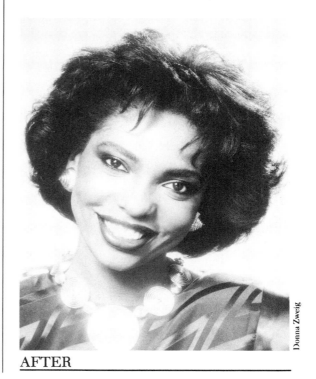

Donna Zweig

AFTER

Kim Hankin

Age 31
New York, New York
Commercial real estate broker
"I look more like myself now,
and much more professional."

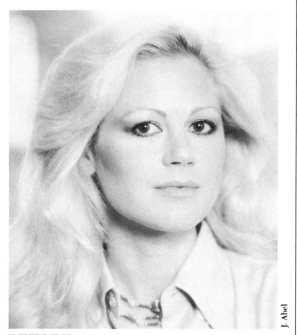

BEFORE

Kim is one of that rare breed, a native New Yorker, born and raised in Manhattan. She was educated at Riverdale Country Day and continued on to Wellesley. When she first came to see me, she was still sporting the hairstyle she'd worn her senior year of college . . . a decade earlier. Over the years, her natural blonde hair had started to darken and as it did, Kim tried highlighting it at first, then did more and more to make it lighter and lighter. She told me she kept remembering the blonde color she'd had as a child. But in an attempt to recapture that shade, she'd overbleached her hair to the point where she was headed for real trouble. Her shoulder-length style was not only out of date, the hair itself was becoming strawlike and very fragile. Because she's such an organized and meticulous young woman, Kim couldn't stand seeing a shadow of regrowth at the roots of her overly blonde hair, so she was having it retouched every ten days!

"I was spending a fortune," Kim exclaimed. "But that was the least of it. I run in Central Park before work every morning and when I get home, I wash my hair then blow it dry at fifteen hundred watts to speed things along. Even so, taking care of my hair after my run was taking so much time, I was thinking of discontinuing the exercise because of the hassle with my hair afterward."

"That's crazy," I told her. "Your hair shouldn't be *limiting* your life-style, it should be enhancing it."

When I looked at Kim, my first thought was "too much." Her hair was too blonde, and suffering from too much exposure. Her eyebrows were too dark, making her face look stark, and her cheeks were too pink. Her hair simply wasn't providing a beautiful frame for her very beautiful face. If Stephanie Tucker, our previous make-over, needed the lights turned *up* on her looks, Kim needed them to be turned *down.* I could imagine what Kim looked like in college, the girl of the year, the one everyone on campus wanted to know. But when I met Kim, she looked very pale, very drained, and very washed out.

I said "Kim, you should look rich, glowing, soft and exciting! Right now you look like a photograph that has been overexposed, with too much light on the subject. I want you to look like you're about to be photographed in natural, warm sunlight, not as if your face and hair have a floodlight trained on them."

"Oh, Leslie," she responded, "I know just what you mean. I feel as if I epitomize that saying about TV anchorwomen, you know, they don't get *older,* they just get *blonder.*"

I had another concern about Kim's image, and that had to do with her professional life. As a commercial real estate broker, she regularly handles major transactions that involve millions of dollars. Although Kim is a natural beauty, the bleached-blonde look had begun to predominate instead of a look of elegance, responsibility, and competence. Once Kim started talking shop, you realized she knew her business inside and out, but the visual image she was projecting wasn't consistent with her professional skills. I felt she would benefit from a new look that would bring her natural beauty and her business life into a closer harmony. I wanted her to look confident, so she would inspire confidence in her clients.

This young woman now looks as if she grew up in a fine home with refined taste, beautiful clothes, good jewelry, and treasured antiques, which describes Kim's background to a T. She reminds me of a young Grace Kelly with her aristocratic features and perfectly flawless skin. Kim has a born-in-the-bone elegance about her that is her birthright and it deserved to be reestablished. She'd almost lost it with hair that had become too light and had gone over the line, but to me, this softer, richer look is what Kim is all about.

"I look more like myself now," Kim said when we finished, "and much more professional."

To bring Kim's looks back into elegant focus, I deepened her hair to a sandy blonde shade, not pink and not yellow, but a light toffee color that suits her perfectly (see chapter 12, Permanent Hair Coloring). When blonde hair is pushed too far, it can assume the cotton-candy look middle-aged women had in the 1960s, and that look was entirely wrong for our elegant Kim. What I envisioned for her was beautiful blonde hair that, when stirred by the breeze, would riffle a little to show a deeper blonde underneath. The light should bounce off Kim's hair and reveal softness and a fresh beauty at the same time. Kim is a highly professional real estate broker, but she is also a friendly, warm person with a wonderful, understated sexiness. I wanted to bring those characteristics to the fore, which is just what I believe we managed to do.

As for a new cut, we trimmed off all the extra hair that had been hanging down over Kim's shoulders and brought the length up to a point where the hair would curve gently against the sides of her neck. I wanted a fuller, more luxurious look to Kim's hair, and since she's got plenty of it, we trimmed the top layers into soft bangs to add an extra bit of flattery to her face. This is a very versatile style for Kim. It can be tied back for sports, worn full and smooth at the office, then swept up for evening. In other words, there are no limitations to what Kim can do with this style, which is exactly right, considering her sports activities, her business, her charity benefits, and her social life.

Once we adjusted Kim's hair color and created a frame for her face so everything wouldn't look as if it were running together, there was very little adjustment that had to be made with her makeup. Her new toffee-blonde shade "opened" her eyes more so you could really see the gray and green flecks in the blue. We lightened her eyebrows and used just a smudge of gray-blue eye shadow plus a touch of liner to bring out

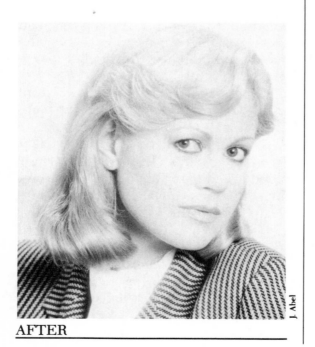

AFTER

J. Abel

her big eyes. A wash of pure beige foundation smoothed out her skin tone and finally a clear-but-true coral lipstick enhanced her warm smile.

Kim needs very little color in her office wardrobe. She can do beautifully with neutral separates—silk blouses, skirts, and jackets in ivories, grays, camels, and beiges. Her new hair color and light eyes create a pretty color impression even if she's dressed in no color at all! And if she likes, Kim can splurge on color for evening with deep sea greens or corals.

As we finished Kim's make-over I looked at her and said, "You look blonde all over."

She smiled and replied, "I know I do, and I love it." The reaction Kim heard from her coworkers and friends was very strong and very positive. "My own eye had to adjust a little," she told me, "but no one else's did. Everyone keeps telling me how marvelous I look."

That's gratifying for me to hear. I talked to Kim again a few days ago. She reported that her business is booming. She has some other news, too. She's engaged to be married. I can't say her new image was responsible, but let's put it this way: It couldn't have hurt!

3

The Action Years

If you're in your thirties you're probably one of the busiest women in the world. No matter what your circumstances, you're working full time and then some. If home management is your job, your children demand your time and taxi services, your husband looks to you for companionship, support, and help in his professional life, and community programs depend on your volunteer hours for their success. Working women don't find it unusual to start their business days with a breakfast meeting, then finish at an industry dinner fourteen hours later. Many women this age juggle family, career, and travel schedules, any one of which would be considered a full-time job. And although they may have an extra set of car keys stashed in the garage, a copy of important telephone numbers taped to the kitchen cabinet, or an extra pair of panty hose tucked into an office drawer, what they *don't* have is any extra *time*.

The outside pressures on a woman in her thirties are enormous. She's constantly trying to meet everyone else's expectations of her, and so plans every single hour of her day so she doesn't waste a minute. She may feel it's selfish or extravagant to spend any time on herself; consequently, the woman she sees in the mirror usually looks exhausted. What she may not realize is that while she's not letting anyone else down, she's giving herself very short shrift, and the chances are she's fallen into a tremendous rut with her looks.

If you are one of these women, the single most important thing you can do for yourself is to carve a few hours out of your schedule for *yourself*! You must replenish your energies and give yourself some of the same care and attention you lavish on everyone else. Responding to other people's demands on your time can be very rewarding and make you feel you truly make a difference in their lives. But if that giving is at the price of constantly ignoring how you look, both to yourself and others, you'll begin to resent those demands over time, and you'll start getting angry, first at them, and ultimately at yourself. Believe me. I hear anger all the time during consultations from women who have postponed and postponed paying any attention to themselves. I want you to take some time *right now* for yourself. Don't waste the gift of your own existence by submerging yourself into other people's lives. Celebrate being the beautiful woman you are in your own right!

I don't want to hear, "But, but, but. . . ." Saying you're too busy or too tired is just a cop-out. *Everyone* is busy or tired, or both. The difference is that some women take the initiative, become assertive, and *do* something about their looks so they can be the best they can be. You can take that action for yourself, too. The payoff is having a polished, finished look as the result. If you say, "I'll do it tomorrow," you'll be too tired when tomorrow comes. Start doing something that makes you feel good about yourself *today.*

Your thirties are no time to sacrifice your good looks or to be *almost* happy with your life. Most likely you already have a good idea of yourself and your best looks. *Clarify* that beauty. These are the years to show yourself off as the beautiful wife, pretty mother, attractive career woman. Enjoy this time. And have some *fun* with your image.

If you've been highlighting your hair in the last few years, take the next step and become a beautiful, shimmering blonde. If you've found those first few strands of gray, either love them or lose them. A rich chestnut brown might suit you perfectly. If your hair has begun to look dull and boring (which can make you *feel* dull and boring), do something about it. How about an exciting auburn? The "action years" are the time not only to *be* active but to *take* action. And the time you devote to yourself now will pay you back tenfold when you're in your forties!

For right now, though, I want you to look as if you really know who you are and love the way you look. This is the time to wear clothes that fit you perfectly, in fabrics that feel good. It's the time to fill your home with things you like looking at and that are a statement of your good taste. And it's the time to give yourself a boost on a regular basis, to keep your looks moving forward with the rest of your life.

You'll find that taking a few hours for yourself is not that difficult to do: a good cut every four to five weeks, refreshing your color, whether every month or once every three to four months, a good perm three or four times a year. All you have to do is to make *yourself* part of your organization plan. You can do it. And it will make a tremendous difference in how you feel. It will do wonders for your psyche, how you view your world, and how you are viewed by everyone else. Taking a small amount of time to pat yourself on the back and say to yourself, I *deserve* this and I'm going to have it, truly changes your outlook and makes you look like the confident, self-assured, great-looking woman you know down deep you really are.

Gail Kislevitz

Age 34
Ridgewood, New Jersey
Wife, mother, consultant
"This is the best I've ever
looked!"

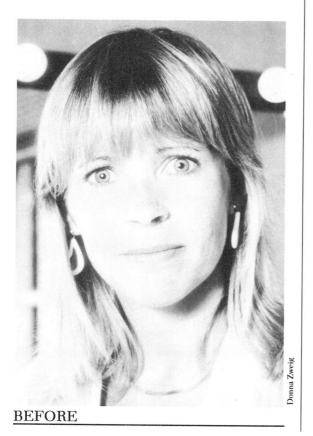

Donna Zweig

BEFORE

Handling as many make-overs as I do for magazines, on television, and in my salon, I've often heard the comment, "She was really so attractive to begin with, how could you go wrong making her over?" It may be absolutely true, but that remark misses the point. I'm not trying to show off *my* skill doing a make-over. I'm trying to help that particular woman realize her greatest beauty potential. If *she* looks in the mirror and doesn't think she looks good, no matter how many *other* people tell her how pretty she is, she won't believe it or, more important, won't *feel* it or *act* beautiful. I want to give every woman I work with clear-cut evidence of how radiant she can look. I want to make her good looks so *obvious* and glorious that even the woman who may have begun to feel like an ugly duckling will see herself as the swan she truly is. And although some make-overs are dramatic, many other times all I have to do is to "point up" a woman's own natural good looks.

Gail Kislevitz is a perfect example of a pretty young woman with natural good looks, but she needed some help to snap them back into focus. And she was aware her looks were beginning to slip. Gail had worked for the international department of a New York bank for several years, then decided to stay home with her children full time. "They were growing so fast," she told me, "that I wanted to spend as much time as I could with them before they were gone, and to me that meant when they would be starting school." Gail submerged herself in suburban life and was pleased with her decision to do so. At the same time, she knew how easy it would be to let her looks slide, because she wouldn't be starting each day putting on makeup, stockings, and a business suit to commute to her office. Nonetheless, she was determined to maintain her polished looks. But schedules, priorities, and *life* being what they are, her resolve faded as she was swept up in car pools, school lunches, committees, meal planning, the works. She was aware she wasn't looking her best but was brought up short when her husband commented, "You're losing it, honey. You don't even dress up much when we go out."

"That really made me think," she confided to me. "I know I'm looking a little drab. . . . I may have forgotten how I used to look. But since my son Elijah is already in second grade and Anna starts kindergarten next fall, I figured it's time for me to get back in touch with myself. And my career. I really need some help right now because I'm going back as a part-time consultant with the bank I used to work for. I'd like to reestablish some of my former professional polish."

Gail's hair had grown a bit too long and, because it's so fine, was beginning to look wispy around the edges. It was dragging her looks down because it had no freshness, excitement, or *swing*. Her skin needed some help, too, specifically more moisturizing and protection, since Gail is athletic and spends so many hours outdoors. And, of course, she was wearing little if any makeup. A quick swipe of lipstick now and then was about it, which left her incredible blue eyes with no frame around them.

———

Gail's natural, sunny glow now shines out in all its glory. Warmth just pours out of her eyes. Looking at her, you really want to talk to this beautiful young woman, to get to know her better. She looks *happy*, vital, pleased with herself and her life, because that's the way she feels now. Her own reaction was "Wow! This is the best I've ever looked!" Gail didn't need a drastic change, just a little "turning around." That was all that had to be done, and so that's all we did.

We started by trimming her fine hair to give it more volume, versatility, and bounce. At this length she can simply finger-dry it at home, take a few minutes to blow it dry if she's going to the office, or smooth it back for evening. Gail loved the idea of not having the same predictable style every day and being able to vary her after-shampoo routine to suit her schedule.

To brighten her naturally dark-blonde hair we added highlights to make it look sunnier, warm, and inviting (for how-to, see chapter 11, Highlighting Your Natural Color). For Gail, it was simply a matter of *complementing* her natural color. Giving her a shade that looked as if we were adding another color to her own blonde would have been much too much. I wanted her still to be a natural blonde but lighter, softer, prettier, and with more sunshine. Gail is an energetic, outdoor, healthy young woman and that's the way her hair looks now.

As for her skin, it is basically very good, but Gail wasn't protecting it enough. I gave her my lecture on proper skin care, making a particular point of what her skin would look like in ten or twenty years if she didn't start taking protective steps right now. The routines you set up for yourself in your thirties show up in your forties and fifties. Consequently, to maintain her good skin, Gail should *never* go outdoors without a good sunscreen. Even further, there are many light foundations these days that contain sunscreening elements. Using one of them *over* a regular sunscreening product for extra protection is a very good idea and one I recommended to Gail. And although Gail should protect her skin, she should never look as if she's wearing a lot of makeup, so we simply dotted a light, sunscreening foundation just across her nose and cheeks to even out her skin tone.

Color on Gail's face should not be too vivid or strong, since her sunny good looks convey enough of a color impression on their own. The lip color we used is fresh and vibrant, but not harsh. If she likes, she can always go brighter for evening. As for her eyes, this is the blue other women have to wear tinted contact lenses to achieve, and Gail was born with them. To make sure they would really stand out as one of her most beautiful features, we used a smoky gray eyeliner and shadow

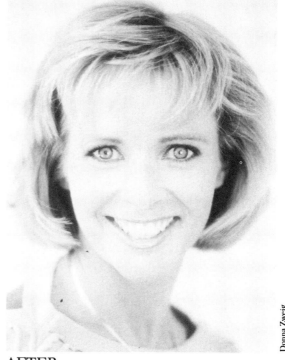

Donna Zweig

AFTER

to dramatize their brilliant blue color.

When we were all finished, Gail commented, "You know, it's amazing how looking drab and unpositive can reflect in the way you feel. Seeing how good you can look, on the other hand, really affects your attitude. And I can tell you, looking this good, I *feel marvelous!*"

Sandy Thompson

Age 35
New York, New York
Graphic designer
"My looks really fit me now."

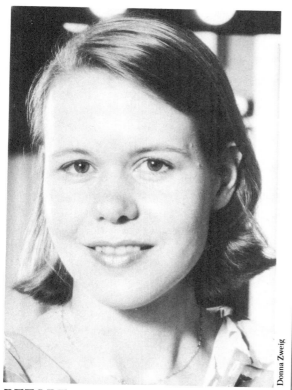

Donna Zweig

BEFORE

Sandy's profession compels her to live in two worlds at the same time. As a graphic designer, she works at home at her drawing board, which is her private, creative life; then she goes out to meet with clients, to deliver her designs, and to discuss new assignments. That's her public life. And although she's enormously successful with her work, she told me she felt her looks had become straggly around the edges. She admitted she'd not been bothering much with her appearance, and yet she felt that she should be looking more professional when meeting with clients. I had to agree with her assessment on all counts.

At home alone sitting at a drawing board, Sandy could wear any old things, pull-on pants, sweatshirts, lumpy sweaters. Her hair could be less than fresh and she certainly didn't need any makeup to work with a T square. The challenge for her was to suit up for her public appearances. What had happened over a period of time, however, was that Sandy had let herself drift so far into the private-time, anything-goes look that getting dressed for her outside appointments had become a bigger and bigger leap for her to make. She simply began to abandon the effort almost entirely.

When she came to see me for her first consultation, Sandy looked as if she had just stood up from her drawing board. She'd washed her hair that morning, but it still looked dull and lifeless. Her hair color was run-of-the-mill mouse brown with no zip or brightness to it. And although Sandy was in no way a drab person, that's the way she had begun to look, at least from the neck up. The day I met her she was wearing a very brightly printed blouse. "Do you wear bright colors like that all the time?" I asked her.

"Well, I've started to lately," she responded. "I guess I feel they pick me up a bit." From what I could see, Sandy was attacking her dull looks on the wrong front. It wasn't a bright blouse she needed, but a whole new, sharper image for herself.

I felt Sandy should integrate her looks more fully so that she'd not only look good at the drawing board (even if *she* were the only one looking at herself), but be able to dress for an outside appointment in no time flat. Working at home, as many of my clients do, you have to be very, very organized. If you don't start your day promptly as soon as the alarm goes off, then meet your daily deadlines, you get so far behind that you never catch up with yourself. And you must use every minute well. Being aware of this from her own experience, Sandy agreed that a new hairstyle that could bridge the gap between her two different worlds would be ideal. Taking less time to get ready for an outside appointment became a definite objective in our makeover. Even further, I felt that since Sandy is a graphics expert, she should have a strong projection of deliberate design about herself, too! I sensed that she could and should be wearing a look that was striking, sophisticated, and even avant garde!

Would you hire this woman to design graphics for you? I would! Sandy now personifies the visual arts. There's nothing tentative or mousy about her looks now. They're bold, definite, and yet very soft and pretty.

There's a deliberate sense of design to the asymmetric cut we gave Sandy's hair: much shorter on one side, fuller and longer on the other. That asymmetry makes use of a classical design element that Sandy understands, is comfortable with, and happens to look terrific wearing. And although there is a geometrical concept in this cut, there are no hard edges to it. The curved outline and soft fringe brushed across her high forehead are very flattering.

"It's so exciting to see myself this way," Sandy exclaimed when she saw herself in the mirror. "My looks really fit me now."

Cutting her hair shorter than she'd worn it in years not only gave Sandy a more stylish look, it took away some of the childishness her old, very basic style had been projecting. And most important, her new hair color revved up her looks so the mousy brown she used to have is nothing more than a dim memory. I didn't feel Sandy's hair should look *too* blonde, however, so we simply highlighted her hair using a "cool" blonde shade to keep things very subtle (see chapter 11, Highlighting Your Natural Color, for details on how to do this yourself). To make the most of her green eyes and pink skin, I chose Moonbeam Blonde for highlights, then scattered a few extra ones across the top to play up the fullness on one side. This adds drama to Sandy's looks and produces a light-suffused frame for her face.

Although we kept Sandy's hair color soft and subtle, we felt we could use lots of color on her face, because she is so comfortable with painting in many different palettes. Blues and violets were perfect for her eyes (she later told me she's experimenting with wine shades now, too). Strong pink went on the lips with a little gloss on top to give Sandy a look of freshness. Also, again because Sandy understands art so well, we used some shading powders to contour her cheeks and define her jawline for a more "sculpted" effect.

As soon as we finished Sandy's makeover, she left the studio to go on several appointments she'd scheduled for that afternoon. She called me the next day to say, "The reaction was incredible! One client said, 'Sandy, I've never seen you in makeup.' The irony is that I *always* wore it, but I guess the overall effect was so low-key that no one really noticed. What really surprised me, though, was that although I felt *very* blonde, no one else commented on the change in my hair color! It was so subtle and fits me so well, that no one else picked it out as the reason why I suddenly look so good." I loved hearing that. It meant Sandy's new hair color was a total success. It made her look pretty and more dynamic, but people noticed Sandy, not her hair color.

Sandy came into the salon recently for a touch-up and told me that the maintenance on her new cut is a snap. "It's so

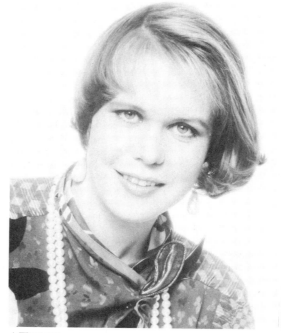

AFTER

Donna Zweig

easy, that even when I got caught in the rain the other day, I just finger-dried my hair between appointments, kept right on going, and it *still* looked good."

I'm delighted Sandy is so pleased with her stylish new looks and with herself, and that she finds keeping up her new image is so manageable. Can you see why I love doing what I do every day? It is so gratifying for me to help a lovely young woman like Sandy redesign her image of herself.

Patricia Bloom, M.D.

Age 35
Hastings-on-Hudson, New York
Wife, mother, physician
"I'll never go back to wearing barrettes!"

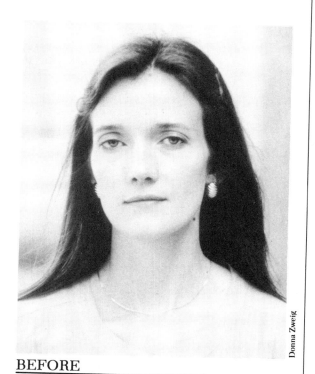

Donna Zweig

BEFORE

Talk about tight scheduling! Patricia is a young woman who has managed to cram a tremendous number of accomplishments into her life. Married in her early twenties, she graduated from medical school, completed her internship and residency, then joined the full-time faculty of Albert Einstein College of Medicine, all by age twenty-seven. Since then she's continued to teach and care for patients. She has had two children in the last six years and commutes every day from a beautiful suburb north of New York City.

I first met Patricia while doing makeovers for the "Good Morning America" television show. When she walked into the studio, I thought she might be a model. She has that long, lean look and stands five feet, nine and a half inches tall without heels. As we talked, I was stunned to learn that not only was she not a model, but she was a doctor specializing in internal medicine and geriatrics. Her looks certainly deceived me!

It was easy to see where Patricia had cut corners in her tight schedule. It was on her own beauty regime. She looked as if she sometimes went months without having her hair trimmed. Further, it appeared to me that she'd scrubbed her face that morning, washed her hair, then yanked it back into two barrettes to get it out of the way as fast as possible. And yet here is a beautiful young woman with gorgeous bone structure, fabulous blue-green eyes, and wonderful hair! She had everything going for her, like a blank canvas begging to be painted.

As we talked further, I discovered that Patricia was moving up in her career. She's just been named director of curriculum development in geriatrics at the hospital. This meant she would not only be assuming more responsibility in her work, but becoming more visible at the same time. I felt she could certainly look more authoritative. People are constantly turning to her for decisions and I wanted her to look as if she could handle all of them. There was a more subtle aspect to what I envisioned for Patricia, too. At first impression, I thought she looked overly strict, yet, talking to her, I found a very warm, caring person. I felt she should look more approachable. I wanted her friendliness to come across immediately.

Teaching and caring for patients means that Patricia spends hours and hours indoors. Yet when you think of "health," you think of sun, brightness, and vitality. A sense of vibrancy was missing in Patricia's appearance, and certainly a lack of color and energy. She had been dressing in neutral colors because they look "professional," but I felt the no-color approach had begun to drab down Patricia's natural beauty. I wanted her to project more vitality and to feel so great about herself that her enthusiasm would spill over into the hours she spent with patients. And, of course, the barrettes *had* to go!

Patricia Bloom, M.D., now has a brand new, *colorful* image. As we finished she said to me, "This is an incredible up." Later at the hospital, one of her patients told her, "Dr. Bloom, I feel better just looking at you."

Our starting point in Patricia's makeover was to create a stronger color definition to her hair, which she had referred to as "dishwater brown." We warmed up the brown with an application of permanent color in a sunny, golden brown, then sprinkled just a few highlights through the hair for an extra glow, but made them so fine that they simply added an extra shimmer to her new, sunny look (see chapter 12, Permanent Hair Coloring, and in particular the section called Highlighting Permanently Colored Hair). I loved the idea that every time Patricia entered a classroom, she'd look as if she were bringing the sun in with her.

Patricia's long hair had made her look too juniorish, and emphasized the length of her neck, but in a negative way. A swanlike neck is one thing, a crane is a bird of a different feather. And although Patricia should *never* have short hair (it would be too delicate for a woman who can go eye-to-eye with a six-foot-tall man), her haircut needed some definite reshaping. We cut it to the point where it would still be long enough to balance her height, but short enough to graze the tops of her shoulders and swing free. And since this doctor's time is so tightly scheduled, we didn't do anything involved or tricky with her hairstyle that would require elaborate maintenance. Both her color and cut are very direct and don't need to be fussed with to keep looking good, a consideration Patricia appreciates.

The minute we warmed and lightened her hair, the glow of color began to enliven Patricia's pretty face. The slightly sallow look her skin had developed was eliminated with apricot blusher, and a coral lipstick brightened her smile. Our makeup artist could hardly wait to go to work on Patricia's blue-green eyes. To make the most of their beautiful color, he used eye-shadow colors in forest green and neutral gray, then drew the eyeliner wide to make her eyes look bigger and more open. Several applications of mascara finished her look.

The way you see Patricia Bloom in her After photo is the way I envision her going out to dinner with her husband. Dressed in a bright, long jacket for color impact and to dramatize her height, she looked absolutely stunning. By coincidence, the day we worked with Patricia was her thirteenth wedding anniversary and she was meeting her husband for dinner that same evening. She told me later, "When he saw me come into the restaurant, he did a double take. He really loved the way I looked." *My* guess is that he saw her in a brand-new light, literally and figuratively!

For the classroom and personal contact with patients, Patricia toned down her makeup, but continued to wear much more than she had before. I firmly believe that once you know how sensa-

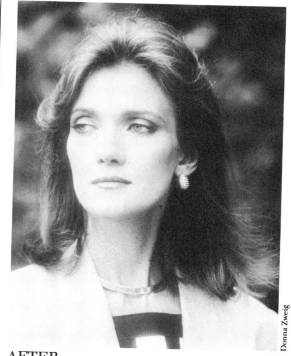

AFTER

Donna Zweig

tional you *can* look, you can always edit your image to suit yourself or your activities. But it's important to see the full picture first. And once you've learned how to maximize your own beauty potential, you're not apt to go back to settling for less. As Dr. Patricia Bloom puts it, "I'll never go back to wearing barrettes!"

Melissa Thornton

Age 33
Trumbull, Connecticut
Entrepreneur, real estate
developer
"I feel very, very elegant."

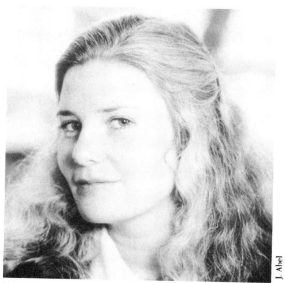

BEFORE

J. Abel

My guess was that while Melissa Thornton might have had brown hair at some earlier point in her life, there was a history of premature gray running through her family. That would be the only logical explanation for a young woman Melissa's age (only thirty-three) to have gone so gray so quickly. "That's true," she confirmed during our first consultation. "Several women in my family went gray while very young. In fact, I started noticing the gray in my own hair when I was only nineteen and a sophomore in college." And while premature gray can look very intriguing on a young woman, I felt the gray Melissa was sporting wasn't doing a *thing* for her looks. To the contrary, it was washing her out and making her look *tired,* when, in fact, she is a dynamic young woman at a most exciting point in her life.

Melissa earned her MBA degree at Dartmouth's prestigious Tuck School of Business Administration. She'd spent several years in corporate life "paying her dues," as she put it, then went to a small market-research company, all the while working toward her ultimate objective of going into her own business. Now every one of the skills she developed in those corporate years is being brought into play. She has, indeed, started her own business building and renovating houses. The avocation she pursued while in the corporate world is now her primary profession. And she's off to a terrific start: She already owns, on her own or in partnership, seven building lots, two income properties, and two houses that are ready for renovation.

Melissa is a flat-out dynamo and her gray hair just didn't fit the rest of her life. Further, I felt the gray made her look a little too formal and cold, when in reality Melissa is extremely outgoing, friendly, and very funny. She has a great sense of humor about herself and everything around her. She's a joy to talk to and spend time with. But all that wonderful warmth and energy were missing from her looks.

This is a woman who meets with a tremendous variety of people in the course of a normal day. She may start her morning with an appointment with a bank officer to discuss a mortgage or to float a loan. From there she'll be meeting with foremen on various construction sites, then go on to review colors, fabrics, and furniture with an interior designer or oversee the installation of new windows in one of her rental buildings. She needs *versatility* in her looks, not the limitations I felt her gray hair was imposing on her. And since so many of her business decisions concern themselves with esthetic judgments, I wanted her to look as if she were applying some of her wonderful taste to *herself.* I wanted her to create a more *positive* impression on the people she meets, not to look like a country girl with no sense of style or with an I-can't-be-bothered-with-it look to her hair.

Melissa Thornton now looks like a woman of substance, a polished professional who radiates warmth, energy, and confidence. If I were her architect or one of her foremen, I'd take one look at her and say to myself, "I'd better do this right, get it done on time, and stay within the budget, too!" And although Melissa's new looks both project and inspire confidence, she certainly doesn't look cool, remote, or formidable. To the contrary, she has an open, inviting look that encourages people to relate to her, both in business and in her personal life. Now she can go from a construction site to a candlelight dinner with perfect ease.

To produce Melissa's casual-but-cared-for look we started by giving her a new cut that would restore some of the natural bounce to her hair. Melissa is tall, vital, and has a full face with wonderful bone structure. She needs hair that fully frames her face in a style that *moves.* She's not the type of person to have every single hair in place at all times. There should be a sense of freedom and energy to her hair.

First we layered and graduated the hair across the top to release all the weight that was literally depressing her hair, then continued graduating the rest of the cut so at its longest it would still clear the collar of any blouse or jacket she might be wearing. This is a versatile, flattering style for her that lifts away from her face and frames those wonderful cheekbones and beautiful eyes.

Because Melissa's natural color had been in the honey-brown family, that's what we decided would look best on her, but with more sparkle and life to it. Using permanent color, which is the best choice for a woman with this much gray, we tinted her hair a light golden brown, then picked out just a few highlights across the top to give her hair a little extra sunshine (see chapter 12, Permanent Hair Coloring). Once we established this warm, glowing shade, Melissa's hair began to look silky and soft, a far cry from the coarse, standoffish gray she used to have. And the golden quality of her hair color gave us our color cue for her makeup.

We carried out Melissa's new sunny look with peachy and coral shades for her skin. We evened out her complexion with a warm beige foundation, then ran a light apricot blusher not only over her cheeks, but all around the edges of her face to give her even more of a warm glow. Eyeliner and eye shadow are both in a deep teal blue to set off her wonderful gray-blue eyes. And a light but clear peach lipstick makes the final point in her new, colorful image.

"I feel very, very elegant!" Melissa exclaimed as we finished her make-over. "I really feel like a star." Melissa left the salon floating on air. When I saw her again a few months later, I asked her how she liked living with her new look. She told me, "It's an incredible boost for me. I can't believe that changing my self-image could have had such a tremendous effect on my life. Because I feel so elegant, I've really developed more energy and have made tremendous strides in my

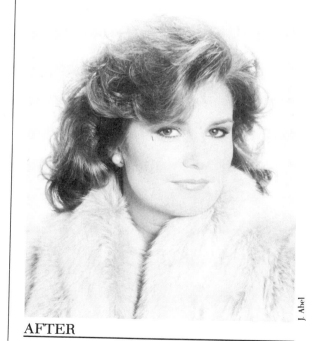

AFTER

J. Abel

new business. I've decided to go on a diet. I figure that if I can look this good at *this* weight, I'll look even better thinner."

It's been a year now since I first met Melissa. She still looks marvelous and, at twenty-seven pounds lighter than she was, even more sensational than she did in her After photo.

4

"What I planted in my life is now blooming and I'm beginning to have more time to myself."
—Sandie McCarthy

Time to Invest in Yourself

It's when my clients move into their forties that they seem inclined to take a close look at their lives. Most women this age are able to see the results of what they began in their twenties, in their children, career, or volunteer projects. It's also a time when many women literally take another look at themselves and ask, "Is this how I want to look at this point in my life?" The forties are a fascinating time, because there's an instinctive urge to take a deep breath, reassess where you are right now, and ask yourself, Is this where I want to be?

For the woman who married straight out of school and had children right away, there's a realization that the kids are now out of the house most of the time, at school, college, or starting their own careers. It's a time to be looking at where *her* life is going next. The woman who has been working for twenty or so years, whether married or single, usually takes a very close look at her career at this point, too, not only to evaluate her progress, but to ask herself if she's still happy with what she's doing. Are the demands of the job still challenging? Or, on the other hand, is she still compelled to work just as hard as she did in her twenties and does she want to keep that pace up indefinitely?

The single most important thing you can do for yourself right now is to realize that it's *your* turn! You've been doing things for others for twenty years or more—husband, children, boss, corporation. Now it's time to be good to *yourself*!

If you've been waiting for the right moment to do something about the gray hair you're not thrilled with, now is the time! If you've always had a hankering to be blonde, do it now! If you're in a rut wearing the same lipstick and eye pencil you wore at twenty-eight, change it to something new and appropriate for a woman in her fabulous forties. If you've always longed for perfect fingernails, set up a series of appointments to get your nails wrapped and manicured regularly. Have you gained too many extra pounds over the years? If you're not happy with the weight, lose it! This is the time in your life to be totally happy with who you are, what you've done, and how you look.

Give yourself lots of credit. As a woman in her forties, you've developed many dimensions to your personality and polished them beautifully. I want you to let your self-esteem shine through now. And I want you to look the best you've ever looked.

Being forty today is equivalent to what being thirty used to be. Today's women in their forties are healthier, more active, and, to my eye, *prettier* than their mothers were at the same age. There's a lot more candor now because women have developed more pride in the age they are and look better than ever. Consider Linda Evans, Donna Mills, Diane Sawyer, and Jacqueline Bisset. They're all delighted to be their age because they know that being forty gives them a definite "edge up." When you're in your forties you've got savvy, self-confidence, and the ability to handle and project yourself in a way you simply couldn't have done in your twenties.

At this age you may find a major shift in emphasis in your life. There may be a new baby on the way. Not one, not two, but three of my clients recently turned forty and became pregnant the same month. You may find yourself separated or divorced and facing life on your own. You may be single, enjoying relationships, other people's children, and suddenly meet the man who makes marriage seem right. Or you may decide it's time for a major career change. Many women who have stayed home with children for twenty years suddenly feel an irresistible urge to get out of the house and back into the mainstream. This usually takes the form of going back to work or making a business out of a hobby. One woman I know took her passion for needlepoint and developed her own mail-order business. Another took the experience she had accumulated from years of chauffeuring kids all over the county and became a successful real estate broker. Another looked at her successful career and decided to take her experience into the classroom. She gave up twelve-hour days at the office in exchange for a three-month summer vacation. Granted, the pay isn't as good but she's happy and comments, "I'm not exhausted at the end of every day anymore."

Whatever your life is evolving into, this is no time to cling to the status quo! It's a time to explore new options, not only in the way you're spending your time, but also in how you look to yourself and others in your world. These are the years to enjoy what you do to its utmost, to surround yourself with people and projects that please you. And it's a time to really *splurge* on yourself, so you will know down deep that you are living up to every particle of potential you have, in your life and in your good looks. Investing in yourself at this age will repay you with handsome dividends for the rest of your life!

Barbara Aversano

Age 40
Lynbrook, New York
Sales administrator
"I'm *amazed* I can look this good."

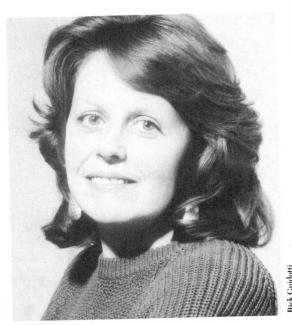

<u>BEFORE</u>

Rick Guidotti

Barbara wrote to me when I was doing make-overs on the "Morning Show" with Regis Philbin. She had just celebrated her thirty-ninth birthday and, as she said in her letter, "I really feel forty coming." The life she'd established for herself in her twenties and thirties had begun falling apart at the seams during the previous eighteen months. To start with, the company for which she'd been working since high school suddenly went bankrupt. That would have been enough of a trauma in itself, but it happened at a very, very difficult time for Barbara. She was taking care of her mother, who was terminally ill, and working two jobs simultaneously to pay for the extraordinary medical expenses involved. She had to find another job, fast. But Barbara herself wasn't feeling that good. She was constantly tired, had little private time of her own, and to relieve some of the pressure, she'd found solace in snacking . . . constantly. As a result her weight had shot up to 205 pounds, much too much for a woman five feet, four inches tall. Yet somehow she had managed to cope, worked part-time as often as she could, and, after her mother died, began to pull herself back together.

By the time I met Barbara, she had already lost fifty-eight pounds! "I know the calorie count of every edible substance on earth," she explained, "so I started eating in a healthy way, concentrating on vegetables and proteins instead of fatty foods. And I made a rule for myself never to eat foods from a package like I did when I indulged in snacks all the time." I applauded Barbara's determination and courage as well as her persistence in losing all that weight. And since she'd already begun to create a new image for herself, I was eager to help her carry that transformation all the way through to her hair and makeup, knowing how fabulous she would look when we finished.

Barbara was starting with some beautiful assets. She has fair, almost translucent, skin and wonderful bone structure. And with her brand-new contact lenses, you didn't have to peer around spectacles to see her lovely gray-green eyes. Those assets gave us a good start, but she wasn't happy with her hair and neither was I. She'd been a redhead as a child, but the gray had crept in over the years. To cover it, Barbara had been using a semipermanent, shampoo-out hair color, but two things had gone awry. Because she'd developed much more gray underneath, the gray was beginning to show through the tint. Also, the shade she had selected had too much yellow in it for her skin and eyes. Hers was a case of sticking to the same method of hair coloring for too long, plus a shade selection that was just off. And on top of everything else, she'd "let her hair go" for several months and the regrowth was really showing. "Oh, dear," Barbara commented, "I've got more roots than Alex Haley!"

Here's Barbara looking bright as a new penny! Her coppery-red hair suits her perfectly and makes the most of her fair skin and wonderful eyes.

To give her hair more vibrance and color personality, we used medium-auburn permanent color that not only covered all the gray effectively, but lent a richer, deeper tone to her red hair (see chapter 12, Permanent Hair Coloring). Naturally red hair like Barbara's should never be permitted to become faded. It's a dramatic color meant always to look vivid and exciting and to impart a definite color personality to the woman wearing it.

With her hair a deeper, richer auburn, Barbara found that her entire appearance started to perk up. Next we looked at the length of her hair, which I felt was too heavy and carried her face down rather than framing it. We cut her hair so it would still be full but shorter and looser. Barbara has wonderful, thick hair and the cut took full advantage of the natural wave in it to make her hair lush and abundant.

Her new hairstyle really accentuated her beautiful complexion. Hers is a true ivory skin, oh so delicate, with the look of fine porcelain. Any makeup used on skin this fair has to be applied very carefully, because it's like painting on a white surface: Whatever color you use shows up immediately. Yet it also offers wonderful choices. Although her hair is auburn, with skin this light, Barbara can go into pinks and cranberries with her makeup colors or she can choose terra cottas and corals. As long as she coordinates cheeks and lips in the same palette (pink with

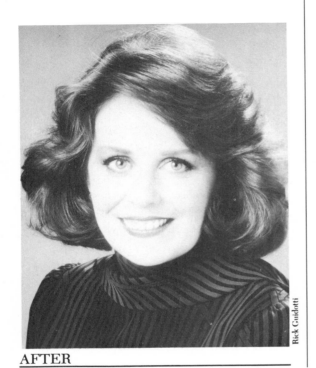

AFTER

Rick Guidotti

berry, peach with coral) she'll look very pretty. But whatever color direction she chooses, cosmetics must be applied with the lightest of hands. Just a touch of blusher, for example, because this type of skin takes color so easily.

The same light touch applies to using color on her gray-green eyes. We used an almost neutral taupe to simply "set" her eyes but not to create an impression of too much additional color. Her hair and eyes together convey enough of a color image on their own!

"I was ready for a total change," Barbara told me as we finished, "but I'm *amazed* I can look this good. Thank you for really caring about me."

Barbara makes it easy to care for her. And from what she's reported since her make-over, her looks continue to have a positive impact on her life. Barbara tells me she feels wonderful in her new classic style because it's as suitable for business interviews as it is for her newly burgeoning social life.

Sandie McCarthy

Age 43
Cypress, California
Wife, mother, model,
community volunteer
"I feel I've been set free!"

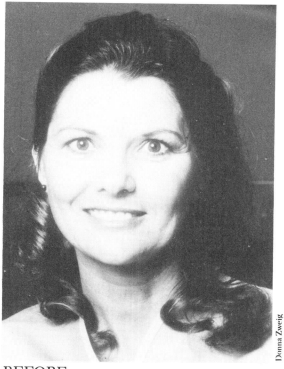

BEFORE

Donna Zweig

Meet a woman who has climbed Mount Fujiyama—twice! Early in her marriage, Sandie and her husband were stationed in Japan while he was in the military service. With her natural curiosity and energy, Sandie was eager to explore the country she was living in. The mountain was there, so she climbed it. That gives you a big clue to Sandie's character— she's a woman of action!

It was also in Japan that her second child was born with a profound hearing disability. In many ways, the birth of that child not only changed the family's life, but directed how Sandie would spend the next fifteen years. Determined that her child would lead as normal a life as possible, she became his teacher. She taught him how to lip-read and how to talk, a phenomenal accomplishment for both Sandie and her son, considering he has never been able to hear the sound of a human voice.

Sandie's children are now twenty, nineteen, and thirteen. The youngest in this close family is a girl who is starting junior high school. Sandie brought her daughter with her when she came to see me and we gave the pretty teenager a new haircut, but my eye immediately focused on Sandie herself. Beautiful features, I thought, and great skin. But a strong widow's peak was bisecting her face and making it look too heart-shaped, almost like a cardboard cutout. And yet there's nothing at all one-dimensional about *this* woman!

"I know I've had my own life on hold for fifteen years," she told me. "It was necessary for me to do what I felt I had to do. But now I'm ready to go forward. What I planted in my life is now blooming and I'm beginning to have a little more time to myself. I want to get out of looking like I'm still wearing my high school or college clothes. I want to feel feminine, pretty, and my own, wonderful age."

"Amen to that," I said. What I saw in Sandie was a magnificent woman ready to move forward with her life. She has many, many talents, a terrific sense of organization, discipline, and determination. She can handle *anything* she wants to do. I wanted to open up her looks so they would match her new ambitions for herself.

We started with a close inspection of her hair. She'd had a perm a year before, had let it grow out, but hadn't trimmed the ends off yet, so they looked an entirely different color from the rest of her hair, both because of the perm and from exposure to the sun. I liked the lighter look the ends hinted at, compared with the dark regrowth that surrounded her face, making it look heavy and shadowed. But I didn't want the lightness to be a result of damage. Rather, I wanted an overall lighter, warmer, sunnier look to her hair.

Sandie's hair texture is very fine, so in terms of a style I wanted to avoid anything that would depend on curl or overly defined geometry. Her hair simply won't hold up to the weight required for that kind of styling; it would collapse under the strain. What her hair needed

was fullness, amplitude, and *movement* as well as a richer, warmer look all over.

Sandie's life is on the move, and now her looks are in forward motion, too. Lighter hair gives a glow to her complexion and brightens her entire appearance.

We lightened Sandie's hair, both in terms of the color we chose and with her new cut. Once all the old ends were trimmed off, her new light-golden-brown hair took on more natural fullness and bounce. A blunt cut created most of the magic, but just around the edges of the front, we cut a few strands slightly shorter, then highlighted them to frame her face with a sunny, golden aura. (See chapter 12, Permanent Hair Coloring, including the section called Highlighting Permanently Colored Hair.)

Because the cut has the effect of lifting Sandie's hair up and away from her wonderful cheekbones, the strict heart-shaped contour of her face is softened and balanced. The slight asymmetry gives sweep to the style and deemphasizes the strong widow's peak, which, while it can be very attractive and certainly shouldn't be hidden, had tended to dominate Sandie's face. I didn't want to see quite so much of a **V** in the center of her forehead. Instead, I wanted to get right to her eyes and her wonderful complexion.

Sandie has had the good sense to care for her skin over the years, and it shows. Her complexion is clear, smooth, and has beautiful luster. The light-golden-brown hair color lends an additional glow to her skin, making it look radiant and even more beautiful. And the scattering of blonde highlights gives her eyes new sparkle, too. Sandie's eyes are a rich, medium brown with golden flecks. The dark hair she had had around her face had made them look simply dark, period. But as soon as we lightened her hair, her eyes lit up as well.

It wasn't necessary to make Sandie's hair *very* blonde. Most brown-eyed women are better off with dark-blonde to light-brown hair, since anything lighter than that will make their eyes too dense by comparison. That's why for Sandie we didn't go any lighter than a light-golden-brown shade to produce a radiant, flattering frame for her face.

"Light" and "soft" apply to Sandie's makeup, too. A creamy beige foundation, a sheer brushing of blusher, and a soft moisturizing lipstick are all she needs. Eye shadows for Sandie come from the amber/gold/bronze palette. Again, we applied just enough eye color to bring out the natural sparkle in her eyes. We lightened Sandie's eyebrows as well, so they would look much softer.

Sandie's first reaction when she looked in the mirror after we were finished was, "Oh, I love it. I can see *me* shining through." And so you can. Sandie's looks are much more in keeping now with the wonderful, energetic, open, and gentle woman she really is.

Sandie's life has really taken off in the last year. She's become very active in the

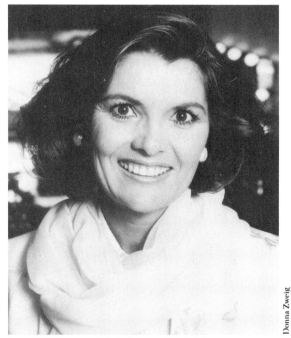

Donna Zweig

AFTER

Assistance League of Long Beach, a California community action group that sponsors a thrift shop, has developed a program for senior citizens, and has established an orthodontic clinic for underprivileged children. She's very involved in the membership committee and is enjoying meeting and working with people she never would have met otherwise.

"This is something I'm not only doing for others. I'm doing it for myself. It gives me a wonderful feeling of satisfaction and accomplishment," she comments.

In addition, Sandie entered a beauty pageant and was named runner-up to "Mrs. California" *and* was voted "Mrs. Congeniality" in the process!

I see Sandie not only as a woman of the 1980s but as a woman of the 1990s. At forty-three, she's experiencing a renaissance in her life and is reaching forward to embrace new ideas, new adventures, new projects, and a new career. She knows that when she spends some time on herself, everyone in her life benefits. "I feel I've been set free!" she told me. "It's hard to believe that simply changing your looks can make such an enormous difference, but it did for me. It's a change that is symbolic of everything else that is happening in my life."

This fall Sandie is planning something else that is symbolic. She and her entire family are taking a trip to Japan. She wants her children to learn more about the Orient, to experience the culture of a different country, and for her middle child, to see the country of his birth. There's a particular part of that trip that means a great deal to Sandie. This time all five of them will be climbing Mount Fuji together.

Kay Bartlett

Age 45
New York, New York
Wire-service feature writer
"I'd forgotten I could look this good."

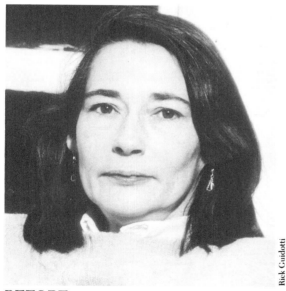

BEFORE

Rick Guidotti

Kay is a pro at meeting deadlines. She's never missed one in her life, which is saying a lot, considering she's been a writer with Associated Press for twenty-one years. That deadline orientation ruled her personal life, too: Shower, dress, and be out of the house every day in ten minutes flat. It's a habit she developed while still in her twenties and "one of the guys" in the pressroom. But while she may have gotten away with that regimen then, I felt she was really short-changing her looks now that she's in her forties. I could understand the urgency of those times when she was speeding to an airport or racing to file a story. But why make rushing a daily routine?

Looking at Kay, I saw a handsome woman. She's a raven-haired beauty with bone structure a model could envy. Since she's naturally tall and very slim, I asked her if she'd ever considered modeling as a career. She told me that in fact she had done some modeling when she was younger, but always loved language so much, she became a writer instead. Nonetheless, you could tell she must have been a knockout in her teens and twenties. At forty-five, however, her looks had slipped, and she knew it. "I've always taken my looks for granted," she told me, "and quite frankly, I never *needed* makeup, so I never bothered learning how to use it. As for my hair, it's always just been there, so I kept it clean and kept going."

Over time, Kay had simply adjusted to looking less than her best. But about the time she was celebrating two decades with AP, she began to feel increasingly restless.

"My professional life has gone beautifully," she said, "and I don't know if I'm in a mid-career crisis or simply feeling middle-aged, but I know something is brewing and that I'm ready for a major change. I just don't know the direction that change will take."

As far as I was concerned, I could see the changes Kay could start with; they were very obvious: She could renovate her hair and learn how to handle makeup! And if changing her looks could help her with whatever other changes might follow, *great.*

The years had dulled the color in Kay's hair. What had been a dramatic dark brown now looked flat and dense. Flecks of gray had started to appear, adding still more drabness to her appearance. The no-makeup policy had contributed, too —negatively. There was nothing colorful in Kay's image, yet there is nothing drab about Kay herself. What I wanted to see in her was rich, rich, rich color! Drama! Excitement! And forget that "poor scribe" look! Here's a natural beauty who should be flaunting her glorious good looks!

Kay no longer looks like "one of the guys." This is a polished professional who has earned her stripes, but is very much in touch with herself as a fabulous-looking woman in her forties.

Kay's dark hair had been falling around her face, covering it up too much and hiding her wonderful features. It's a mistake that's all too common, but when it's made by a brunette, it has particularly dire consequences, because of the shadowing effect it produces. The first thing we did was to give Kay a new cut that drew the heavy curtains back off her face so you could really see who she is— a woman with beautiful eyes and incredible bone structure. Kay's looks are those of a classic beauty and to show them off to their best advantage, her new hairstyle is equally classic, a blunt cut softly brushed to frame her face. In trimming her hair, we made it short enough to swing free of her shoulders and to give the impression of movement and energy.

And I was desperate to revitalize the *color* in Kay's dark hair. When the rich dimension is taken out of a brunette's hair, as happens with age, the brown loses its vibrancy and appears drab and flat. This holds true for all brunette hair and certainly applied to Kay's. To restore the rich dimension to Kay's color, we used permanent hair coloring in a dark cool brown with just a touch of warm coloring, which was all she needed (see chapter 13, Leslie Blanchard's Favorite Salon Formulas).

Because of Kay's natural coloring (dark eyes, fair skin, and dark hair) any little thing she does to her looks will appear to be very dramatic. While we didn't cut her hair that much shorter, nor alter the color of her hair that substantially, the changes we *did* make are emphatic. Kay's natural elegance is apparent, but pointing up her looks with small changes makes all the difference in whether Kay's beauty comes across as understated or simply mute.

As you've seen in several of our previous make-overs, once a woman's hair is lighter or brighter, her skin takes on more light and luster, too. Kay's skin was no exception. Her complexion now looks smoother, pinker, and has more vitality. Shades of mauve, lavender, violet, and mulberry look wonderful against this type of skin, so that's how we chose her makeup colors. Kay's first reaction to her new looks was a long, low, "Wow! I'd forgotten I could look this good."

Kay is an example of an extraordinarily attractive woman who has always had beautiful features and never had to do much with them to look good. Her indifference to her own good looks had finally caught up with her. But now that she's reidentified herself in the mirror, she won't have to go to extreme lengths to keep up her good looks. Even if she's not wearing any makeup (changing flights in Chicago at midnight, conducting an interview by dawn's early light), she'll still look good, because her *hair* will look good and that goes a long way toward maintaining her positive image.

Kay told me a funny story. On her way back from the photography studio (still in full makeup and freshly done hair), she was crossing the street when a man passed her and muttered, "These rich women."

"It took me a minute to realize he meant *me*," Kay laughed. "Then I

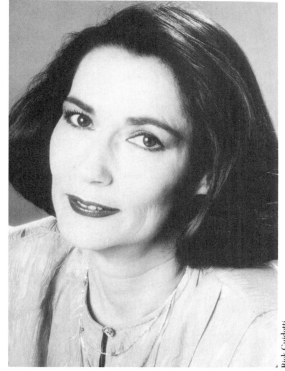

AFTER

Rick Guidotti

thought, It's nice to look rich for a change, even if you're just on your way back to the office."

And there was a lot of kidding from her associates when they saw her. "Who is this woman? Kay Bartlett, star?" But they were *very* impressed. One woman asked her, "What color was your hair yesterday?" She couldn't recall, perhaps because the drab brown was so eminently forgettable!

Kay described her mood after her make-over as "euphoric." "I didn't want to take my new makeup off that first night. I loved the way I looked. I thought, If I can look like this, I can do *anything.*"

She's coming back to the salon for a proper lesson in how to apply makeup, which I feel she can benefit from. When she called to schedule the appointment, she said, "Leslie, you read me like a book. I'm so grateful that you didn't take the changes you made in my looks too far. You called me classic and that's just the way I feel."

Classic, yes, Kay, and very beautiful.

Karin Bardram

Age 49
Essex Fells, New Jersey
Wife, mother of four
"I feel so much lighter!"

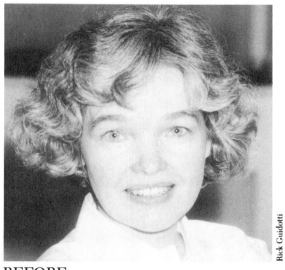

BEFORE

The color picture we took of Karin before her make-over might as well have been shot in black-and-white film. There was almost *no* color in the way Karin was projecting herself. Her gray hair was verging on white, she wore no makeup, and she was dressed in the most neutral shades of clothing. The only reason we didn't waste the color film was her fantastic blue eyes. Not only can you see them in her Before photograph, in person you can see them clear across the room!

Karin wasn't that concerned about her gray hair. She said it didn't bother her. Although she was born in the United States, both her parents are Swedish and she's lived on and off in Europe over the years. She told me, "Perhaps I've absorbed more of the European attitude toward my hair. They attach less importance to going gray."

It was her all-American children who were after Karin to make a change in her looks. "Mom, you're too young looking to have all that gray hair," they kept telling her. Her children range in age from seventeen to twenty-two. The eldest just finished college and three are still undergraduates. I wondered if Karin's kids were on her case because their classmates' mothers looked younger than their mother, but whatever the reason, Karin arrived at my salon one day for a consultation.

The first thing I saw was her gray hair, *then* I noticed Karin. In that flash, I realized her hair was overpowering this great-looking woman. Not only was the gray color washing out her natural beauty, I was bothered by the sheer *volume* of hair you had to get past to see Karin herself. When most blondes go gray (including most Scandinavians) they become dishwatery looking, because the hair texture is so fine. But Karin's gray hair had come in thick and very heavy. She was so unfamiliar with its new texture that she'd had a perm to make it more manageable. But now the perm was growing out, leaving her hair looking coarse and dry. Karin looked as if she were carrying a huge weight on her head, which was pulling everything about her *down* and making her look *tired.* Yet her incredible blue eyes had such sparkle, I wanted to cue her looks to *them,* not to the ton of gray hair she was toting around.

The full-color After photo of Karin's black-and-white image dramatizes the tremendous difference she made in her looks. Usually I can visualize very clearly how a woman will appear when we've finished her make-over, but Karin's After amazed even me! I'd said I felt she needed more *color* but didn't anticipate the extraordinary extent to which Karin could wear color well. Then it dawned on me. Of course, I thought to myself, look at all those bright colors Scandinavians are partial to in their fashion and in their homes—the brightest blues, the vivid reds, the Marimekko marigolds. They use intense color to brighten their

dark days and long winter nights.

On one hand Karin looks very American, but on the other, she shows a spectacular capacity for color that is a real gift from her Swedish ancestry. I loved the fact that she was able to take advantage of the best of both worlds to look so wonderful.

When Karin looked in the mirror, she said, "Oh, I love it. I feel so much lighter!" That was what we had in mind. At some point in her life Karin may decide to go back to gray, but for right now, I didn't find it becoming to her. That's the criterion I always use and wish every woman would use for herself. Loving or losing your gray hair isn't a decision to make because you think you should cover it at a certain age, or should let it go gray because you are getting older. The only important question to ask yourself is, Does my gray look good on me? If it does, keep it! If it doesn't, cover it. Karin's gray was aging her and making her look too reserved, so we changed it. She has plenty of time later to enjoy gray hair, but with college-aged daughters, I thought she'd look better with a wonderful blonde shade closer to the color she had when she was younger, and closer to the natural blonde both her daughters have inherited from her.

The actual color we used on Karin was between light- and medium-golden blonde to give a warmth to her looks and a sunny glow to her complexion (see chapter 13, Leslie Blanchard's Favorite Salon Formulas). In addition, we picked out just a few highlights in the palest blonde shade to make Karin's hair look as if she'd spent the summer in the sun. (See chapter 12, especially the section called Highlighting Permanently Colored Hair.) Besides looking so wonderful on her, hair coloring gave Karin's coarse, dry hair a new, silky quality with lots and lots of shine.

To keep her hair outdoorsy and breezy looking, we trimmed some of the weight off the top, then reshaped the sides where it had become so wide that it was making her face look round. Once we had the cut under control, Karin's perfectly balanced bone structure started to come through and her incredible blue eyes assumed their rightful place as a beautiful focus for her face. Wearing vibrant colors as Karin does so well requires a little extra makeup, so we used a taupe eyeliner for added definition, then followed it up with a rosy-taupe eye shadow. Lipstick is vivid to suit her fashion choices, almost a bright burgundy. But if Karin wishes, she can go into paler pinks for daytime or outdoor sports—a light rosé, for example.

Karin confessed that as good as she thought she looked, it took her at least a week to get used to her new image. I'd consider that right on time, since any woman who was as gray as Karin will need some time to adjust when her looks are changed as completely as Karin's were. Once she'd awakened for a few mornings and seen herself looking like this, though, she really started to appreciate the change. "It's absolutely beautiful," she commented.

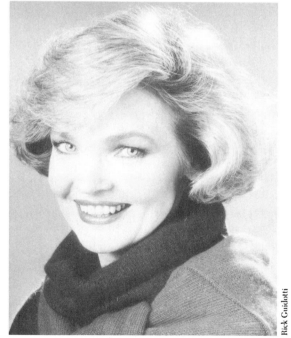

AFTER

Rick Guidotti

Shortly after her make-over, Karin drove down to Virginia to pick up one of her daughters at college, the one who had been the most vociferous about her mother's gray hair. Karin climbed the five flights of stairs in the dorm, wondering all the way why the elevator was out of commission. As she reached the top, she saw why. One of the students had jammed the elevator door to load it up with her luggage and cartons of books. Karin bent down to give the girl a hand, then a third pair of hands chipped in. Karen glanced up and suddenly was eye to eye with her own daughter. There was a moment of dead silence, then an explosion of recognition: "Mom, it's *you*! I never would have recognized you. Oh, you look fabulous!"

If Karin hadn't been getting constant encouragement from her kids, she might not have taken the plunge in changing her looks. Then again, maybe the change was something that down deep she'd been considering all along. She told me, "It was so much *fun*. I had no idea I'd enjoy myself so much or feel so wonderful afterward. I'm sorry I didn't do it sooner. And I'm getting compliments all the time. The one I like best came from my son's girlfriend. She said, 'Mrs. Bardram, I don't know what you did to yourself, but you look terrific.' She didn't say, 'What you did to your *hair*,' just 'yourself.' That's why I feel her compliment was the best of all."

I agree, Karin, you look terrific.

5

"This is wonderful. It's my personal best."
—Lola Fisher

The Good Life

If being forty is fabulous, being fifty is *fantastic!* The fifties are the age of liberation. If you are a mother child-care responsibilities have been substantially accomplished, if you are married or have a special loved one relationships are established, friendships are flourishing, and it's time to enjoy the good life. It's a wonderful time because you can now concentrate on those things that make you feel happiest and are most personally rewarding to you.

Although you may not be a spring sapling, there's plenty of juice still flowing. Some of the most beautiful women in the world are in their fifties: Elizabeth Taylor, Sophia Loren, Audrey Hepburn, Jacqueline Onassis. You may not be able to match measurements with Joan Collins, but give her credit for creating a new image of a sexy woman in her fifties. *Post-menopausal* is a term that sounds hopelessly out of date. Forget it! Did you see Jane Powell on television at the Oscar presentations last spring? Wow! She's as trim and pretty as ever. Didn't Angie Dickinson look sensational? And when NBC was looking for a news anchorwoman recently, they hired Pat Harper, a stunning, accomplished woman in her fifties. See what I mean about "juice"? Most women this age are just on the other side of being halfway through their lives. Statistically, they've got another twenty-five or thirty years ahead. That fact alone should be enough to rev up your engines and get you *really* going. And although it's a good idea to pause and see where your life is at this age, it's no time to relax into the rocker and start reviewing scrapbooks!

The single most important thing you can do for yourself at this age is to identify what makes you happiest, then pursue it with energy, enthusiasm, and verve. Being curious, active, and *involved* is what will do the most for your good looks—that, and keeping your beauty at its highest possible polish.

You'll want your skin to look thoroughly moisturized, just like a flower in full bloom. In addition to keeping your skin protected, you might consider using one of the "cell renewal" skin-care products now on the market. I've seen them make a difference in some women's skin. Makeup looks fresher at this age with a little less color around the eyes but more *definition,* as with a carefully drawn eyeliner. Use a magnifying mirror if you have to, but apply it perfectly. Blusher should be on the light side, too, but keep it north of the tip of your nose and, please, no grinding rouge into circles to affect the "apple cheeks" of a teenager. That's *deadly* on an older woman. As for the lips, a bright, *affirmative* shade is best—neither too dark nor too pale and sappy. As for that seepage of lip color into the vertical creases around your mouth, look for a "dry" finish in your lipstick. There are several brands around now that are described as "antifeathering" that really work. And please, no iridescent anything; it just magnifies any creases your skin may have developed.

With hair color, if you love your gray, *flaunt it*—in a soft, contemporary style that looks as if you could run your hands through it at any moment. No hair-spray helmets, please. If you *feel* younger and more energetic with rich color in your hair, that's your choice! If you've been coloring your hair over the years and want to see what you'd look like totally gray, let your hair grow out and take a look. Most women I know who have done that say, "Oh, no, that's not me," and go right back to a rich flattering color. But if you like it on yourself, *stay* with it. Listen to your own advice to yourself. At this age, it's the best you'll ever get!

By this point, you've developed some wonderful life experiences; now build on them. And *share* what you've learned. Don't be surprised if younger women and men turn to you for advice. After all, you've probably lived through whatever they're going through now and look how beautifully you and your life are turning out!

As you move into your sixties, seventies, and eighties, you may find you're not physically up to as much as you were in your forties or fifties, but that's no reason to shut down your life, roll up the carpets, and abandon your good looks. Resolve to yourself *never* to say, "I'm too old for that." My grandmother was in her vigorous eighties when she went on to greater gardening. My mother is in her seventies now, works part-time, and loves her life. Can you imagine Katharine Hepburn refusing a challenge? Or Barbara Bel Geddes sitting home alone? How about Gwen Verdon, Cyd Charisse, Mary Martin, Ann Miller, Barbara Stanwyck, or Jane Wyman? Do they strike you as women who have resigned themselves to a life of limitations? Scarcely!

This is no time to act *or look* like a little old lady! Hair thinning? Keep it short and fluffy. In terms of color, revel in your gray or keep it a medium shade that's softer than what you had in your forties: softer brown, softer red, not quite so blonde. Too dark will make your hair look even thinner, too light will make it look transparent. As for hairstyling, if you've been going to the same hairdresser for years and that person greets you with "The usual?" find yourself a cute new stylist who wants to try something different with your hair.

The only limitations you have at this point in your life are those you put on yourself. And I don't want you to *look* limited, either. Spend part of every day on your own good grooming. Create some rituals for yourself. Bathe at least every other day with a skin-smoothing body oil. Wash your hair at least twice a week. Trim your fingernails to an even length, whether or not you wear nail polish. If you store your out-of-season clothing in mothballs air them out *thoroughly* before wearing; you'll *smell* old otherwise. And keep the cologne under control. Our sense of smell becomes less acute with age—if you can smell the cologne on *yourself,* it may be too much for everyone else around you. Buy at least one new jacket or dress twice a year, in the fall and again in the spring. If you try, you'll find a way to look current, even on a fixed income. At this age, meeting a friend for lunch in a stunning new outfit speaks *volumes* about you, all of it positive. Get out of the house and out of yourself. Life is too sweet and precious not to enjoy it to the full and to celebrate being the beautiful woman I know you are.

After an entire career based on making changes in women's looks, I have, over the years, come to a few conclusions I'd like to share with you, in case they can lend some perspective. Change is inevitable. Life and time do not stand still. So if you are going to have to make changes anyhow—whether or not you want to—you may as well make them for the better. You may as well *enjoy* the changes life brings and aim them at making you feel your happiest and most beautiful. You see, every day of my life is filled with new beginnings. That's why I love what I do. I want *your* life to be filled with that same ongoing sense of discovery.

Rhoda Friedman

Age 48
Newport Beach, California
Wife, mother, community volunteer
"I've never looked better."

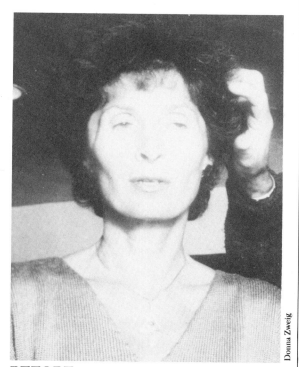

BEFORE

Donna Zweig

Although Rhoda Friedman is still in her forties, she has a running start on living the good life. She married and had her children in her early twenties; now both her children (ages twenty-seven and twenty-five) are married and on their own. At this point, Rhoda and her husband, a dermatologist, have begun to have the time *and* the inclination to pursue their own interests.

I first met Rhoda when I was doing make-overs for the "A.M. Los Angeles" television show and selected her because she looked as if she lived the California life to the fullest, which she does. Her house is near the beach, she enjoys tennis, golf, sailing, and loves to travel. She and her husband plan at least one big trip each year. They've already presented their passports in France, Israel, and Singapore, and there are more countries to come. Rhoda claims one of her hobbies is crossing time zones!

Rhoda is blessed with a wonderful sense of curiosity and constantly reaches out to explore new projects, new cultures, new ways of spending her time. Back when she was thirty and the children were both in elementary school, she wondered what would be involved in going back to school herself for a graduate degree. She found out soon enough and was awarded her master's degree in library science in 1971. She's worked on and off over the years and most recently signed on as a volunteer docent at the Newport Harbor Art Museum, which has a fine collection of contemporary art. She lectures and leads tours of the museum and that was one of the reasons she came in for a consultation. "I'm dealing with the public all the time," she told me, "and meeting new people every day. I'd like to be presenting the best personal appearance possible." But when I asked Rhoda if there were any *other* reason she wanted a make-over, she said, "Yes. Because I'm *curious* to see what you can do with my looks." I was delighted at the prospect of satisfying Rhoda's curiosity, so we got started right away.

On first impression, I thought Rhoda looked older than she really is. She'd taken fairly good care of her skin (probably at the behest of her dermatologist husband) and had a light tan from her outdoor sports. When you looked at her hair color and her complexion *together,* however, they looked "muddy" to my eye. Rhoda had been coloring her hair to cover her almost seventy-five percent gray, but the color she'd used looked too *solid,* and much too dark. I wanted to give her hair more of a play of light, to warm it up a little so you could really see those great cheekbones. She has a Sophia Loren quality to her looks and that's what I wanted to dramatize.

As we age, the hair naturally loses its color pigment and goes gray. To some degree, the skin does the same thing: the rosy complexion of youth fades. So, to keep the skin tone looking warm and healthy, it's necessary to add some warmth to your hair color, even if it's only a little. Since your face and your skin interact with one another, the drab-ber the hair color, the drabber the skin will appear. That's what I saw happening with Rhoda. The hair coloring shade she had been using was one shade too dark and one hundred percent "cool," so there was no warmth or vibrancy to either her hair *or* her face. I wanted to give her lighter, sunnier-looking hair and to make her appear soft and *fresh.*

Now Rhoda looks as if she's stepped out from under a cloud and is enjoying a beautiful California day filled with sunshine. Here's a woman who should never be a blonde—she doesn't have the eyes or the skin to make that color believable on her—but that doesn't mean she can't have golden highlights streaming through her hair to lend a sunny, California *spirit* to her looks.

What did she feel when she first looked in the mirror after our make-over? "Awe," Rhoda said. "I've never looked better. But at the same time I don't feel looking like this is beyond the scope of possibilities for me." Rhoda could see some of the specific changes we'd made in her looks very clearly, but I wanted her to understand everything we did so she could keep this look going on her own.

I explained to Rhoda that the biggest change we made in her hair color was to shift from the cool shade she'd been using to a warm medium brown. That set our color direction and prepared the "canvas" on which we then "painted" golden-blonde highlights. (See chapter

12, Permanent Hair Coloring, including the section called Highlighting Permanently Colored Hair.) We concentrated the highlights across the top of her hair *only,* to add light to the top part of her face and to bring her eyes out more. If you notice, the sides of her hair were kept in the warm medium brown. The reason we did *not* highlight the sides of her hair was that I wanted a slightly deeper shade at that point of her face, to set off her cheekbones in the most dramatic way possible. Keeping the hair slightly deeper at the sides framed her bone structure and transformed this marvelous beauty asset from potential to flattering reality. As for her new hairstyle, it was more a reshaping than a revolution. The hair was left full at the top for extra lift, then tapered closer toward the nape in a carefree, contemporary style.

The changes we made in Rhoda's hair gave us a good start in brightening her entire appearance. To follow through in the same feeling, we adapted her makeup along those same lines. Rhoda's eyes are very deep-set and with her hair darker, they'd looked even darker, deeper-set, and smaller than they really were. We used a light eye shadow in a honey-sand color to bring her eyes forward, give them more sparkle, and make Rhoda look more wide-eyed. After a certain age, strong color becomes less and less important around the eyes. To a great degree, vibrant hair color and a clear lipstick will convey enough of a color impression on their own. What the

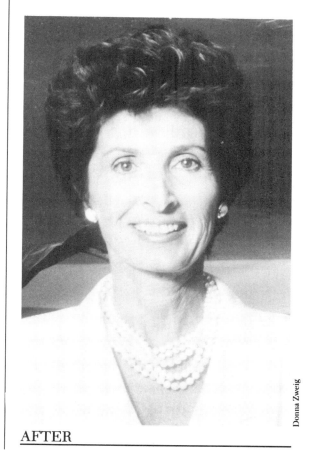

Donna Zweig

AFTER

eyes will benefit from, however, is more *definition.* To accomplish this, we used a soft hickory-brown eyeliner on Rhoda, which gave her eyes that extra bit of expression.

Looking as she does in her After photo, Rhoda could be the president of her own company or mayor of her city. For her sports life, however, she can simply edit the makeup down a little and blow her hair dry a little less fully. Rhoda caught on to that concept right away. "Being aware of the full effect is very valuable. I may not take the time every day to follow every step to the letter, but now that I've seen the full picture, I doubt if I'd go out of the house without *some* makeup!"

"Fresh" is one word that occurs to me looking at Rhoda—and "fashionable," including her accessories. If you're over forty, the single best accessory you can buy for yourself is the longest strand of pearls you can afford. Look how this *tangle* of pearls lights up Rhoda's skin and eyes!

Her husband loved the way Rhoda looked. "Gee, honey, you look just great," he told her. The Friedmans are looking forward to what the good life will be bringing them in the years to come.

"More travel," Rhoda said. "And grandchildren, we hope. And my husband will probably have our first grandchild on a Windsurfer as soon as the baby can walk." Spending part of the good life on a Windsurfer with one of your children's children sounds like a terrific idea, doesn't it?

LaVonne DelCol

Age 51
Chappaqua, New York
Mother, assistant store manager
"Now I feel set for the *next* decade."

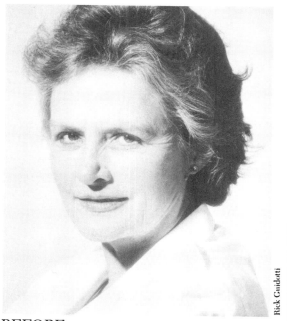

BEFORE

Rick Guidotti

When LaVonne DelCol first came to see me, she wanted a new cut. And, maybe, a little color. She wasn't sure. She felt she needed more of *something*, though. Highlights, perhaps? But one look at her and I thought: *Structure*. She needs structure to her color and more structure to the shape of her hair.

In talking with LaVonne I found that the image she presented to me of being "at loose ends" with her looks was eerily representative of what else had been going on. The primary structure in her life, a marriage of twenty-two years, had ended. On her fiftieth birthday she found herself unexpectedly single. It was a very, very difficult turning point for her and a real crisis. But by the time La-Vonne came to see me, she'd been through the worst part of the adjustment. Her three children (ages twenty-four, twenty-three, and twenty) had been a help. And she'd found work she enjoyed. She's the assistant manager of a shop that specializes in decorator fabrics. LaVonne had already initiated some new beginnings for herself and she was ready to carry that spirit of regeneration through to her personal appearance.

In my professional experience, I've found that making a substantial alteration in your looks is most successful when it's made *after* other big changes in your life. Changing your image while you're still unhappy rarely solves your central problem. But once you're through the transition, have settled down, and feel you're ready for the first day of the rest of your life, treating yourself to new hair color and a new hairstyle can do wonders. Nothing gets you back in touch with the wonderful woman you are *faster* than looking in the mirror and seeing a sensational reflection. Changing your image for the better after a crisis speeds the healing process, retunes your engines, gets you back on track, and helps you set new directions for yourself.

I was seeing too much of LaVonne's past in her appearance. I wanted her to look centered, confident, and ready for all the new beginnings that are in her future. Our starting point was LaVonne's hair. She's a former blonde; as her color faded to light brown she'd tried some highlights to brighten her hair. But as she continued to highlight her hair, it kept getting grayer and grayer so the color was straddling the line between gray and beige and ended up being a rather dingy "greige," and not at all flattering. When I met her, she'd let her hair grow out completely because she was unsure of what else to do. The plain gray wasn't flattering either. Her beautiful complexion had begun to look tired and the gray was draining almost all the color out of her gorgeous blue eyes. At some point in the future, LaVonne might consider opting for sparkling gray hair, but for right now, I felt her gray didn't seem to be going forward with the rest of her life. Her style had grown out, too. It was a little too long, a little too heavy, and had very little shape. LaVonne's hair simply needed a little tender loving care and attention, and so did she!

Here's a perfectly pampered LaVonne. "Oh, I look so much *younger*," she exclaimed. "I like looking like *this* a whole lot more than what I'm used to seeing in the mirror." LaVonne's new sunny appearance is not only more flattering to her than the gray, it makes her seem more competent and authoritative in her business life. Giving customers advice on which colors and fabrics will work well together in a room is something LaVonne does every day. When she went back to work after her makeover, some of her customers didn't recognize her at first, they just knew she looked terrific. Now that LaVonne has organized her personal color coordination so beautifully, I'll bet you a yard of flowered chintz those customers will be seeking out her advice much more often.

Pulling together LaVonne's good looks was a classic example of bringing out what was already there. The shorter cut helped bring back her hair's natural wave, which in turn made her hair look fuller, thicker, and more abundant. The hair coloring not only contributed a beautiful, soft shade but added extra body, texture, and shine, shine, shine to her hair. To produce this particular blonde shade for LaVonne, we mixed a formula of permanent hair coloring that included both warm and cool blonde shades: the warm accent to light up her skin, and the cool to enhance the blue of her eyes (see chapter 13, Leslie Blanchard's Favorite Salon Formulas). To make her face seem less round, we scattered a few pale golden highlights just across the top of her face, to give it a little more height and to light up the eye area.

This hairstyle is very simple and one that LaVonne can handle herself very easily. Minimum maintenance was in the back of my mind when designing this cut because I didn't want LaVonne locked into salon appointments to keep looking good. And there was still another good reason for developing this easy-care style. It's a great cut to have while you're traveling. You see, LaVonne was scheduled to take the trip of a lifetime soon after her make-over. She was leaving for China! I was determined that LaVonne was not going to look as if she were trailing suburbia through the airport in Peking! This smart, contemporary cut will look good throughout any vacation, even after it's crossed the international dateline.

With her soft, pretty blonde hair and very blue eyes, LaVonne doesn't need much color in her makeup for a finished look. To help define her eyebrows, which had faded away a bit too much, we tweezed out the extra strays, then filled in with a light ash-brown pencil, primarily to add more shape to her eyebrows. And to put those beautiful eyes into very clear focus, we used a dark-brown eyeliner and a neutral taupe eye shadow to set them perfectly. Foundation and blusher were kept very light and fresh: a little smoothing out of the skin tone and just a flick of color over the cheeks. Since she has strong cheekbones and a firm chin line, LaVonne can wear a fairly

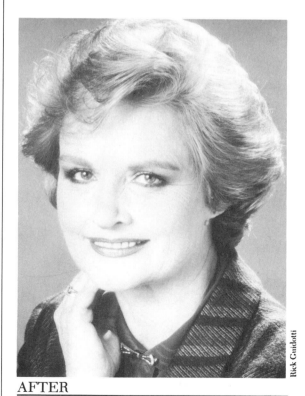

AFTER

Rick Guidotti

deep lip color well; this one is a pretty brown-berry shade.

LaVonne is planning to take some of her new cosmetics with her while traveling. I suggested she take along her own shampoo and conditioner, too. As for a blow dryer, that's up to her. Sometimes when traveling, you're moving at such a brisk pace and having such a good time exploring the country you're in, you want to be able to shampoo, condition, towel dry, and get out of the hotel. That's an option LaVonne now has.

LaVonne told me, "The first few days after my make-over, I found myself doing double takes in the mirror. But I really love my new looks and have become very comfortable with them. Now I feel set for the *next* decade." LaVonne is planning to make at least one big trip a year from now on. She's not only facing the future, she's grabbing at it. I'm glad I could help her get her looks in line with her life and I wish her my warmest bon voyage.

Barbara Levee

Age 56
Cincinnati, Ohio
Wife, mother, stepmother
"This is the best style I've ever had in my life!"

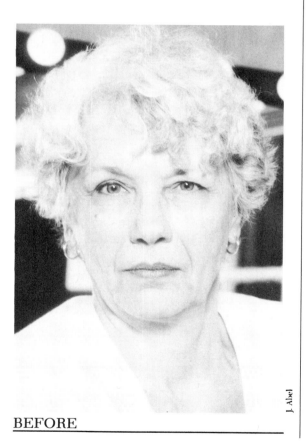

BEFORE

Barbara Levee has made a habit of reaching out for change. She does it the way a flower turns to light, instinctively. She was looking for a new hairstylist when I first met her. She'd had the same one for years but couldn't make him do anything different with her hair. "Just because *he* doesn't want to try anything new doesn't mean *I* don't. I refuse to be in that same old lock-step."

Six years ago, just at the time she was turning fifty, Barbara started a new life. She remarried and gained a new husband, and several more children as well. Between them, Barbara and Joe Levee have eight kids, seven of them daughters! The children are grown now and range in age from twenty-four to thirty-one, but back when Joe's eldest daughter was graduating from college and beginning her job hunt, he gave her a present, a make-over at the Private World of Leslie Blanchard. The Levees were living in Connecticut at the time and to celebrate their daughter's After they made a date to have dinner with her in New York. They took along two of their other daughters and all five of them had a wonderful time. That became the first of several celebratory dinners. Each of the other girls in turn was given a make-over followed by an evening on the town. When I first met Barbara, I felt she was already "family" and could hardly wait to do for her what I'd been able to do for her daughters.

Although Barbara was overdue for everything—a new cut *and* a new perm—I loved her gray hair and felt it suited her perfectly. It was such a beautiful gray, I didn't even *think* of changing it. Barbara had gray hair when she met Joe, she was accustomed to thinking of herself as gray-haired, and was in the habit of *playing up* her gray in her choice of fashion. The only thing I felt strongly about was adding more excitement and sparkle to Barbara's gray. I wanted it to look like beautiful, freshly polished silver.

As for a new hairstyle, I wanted to reverse the downward direction her hair had assumed as it had grown out. With hair this fine, you must keep your appointments for a regular trim or perm exactly on schedule lest your style begin to collapse on itself. What I wanted for Barbara was a look that was uplifting, one that would aim the eye of the beholder up to her cheekbones and marvelous eyes. I wanted her to look confident. Important. I wanted her to really *flaunt* her gray.

Here's Barbara Levee looking totally glamorous and glamorously gray! "Oh, it's great! This is the best style I've ever had in my life," she exclaimed. She could hardly wait to meet her husband and daughters for dinner that evening. It was *her* turn to be the center of attention in what had become the family's ritual celebration.

In polishing up Barbara's gray hair color, we used nothing more than a temporary rinse in the lightest, whitest platinum. Her gray was a pretty shade to begin with, but to keep gray looking as clear and sparkling as crystal, whether you add a rinse or not, you must be sure it doesn't pick up a single speck of yellow. Hair spray can yellow gray hair and so can pollutants in the air, so it's important to keep it immaculately clean. Once shampooed, all you may need to heighten your gray color is the type of temporary rinse we used on Barbara (see chapter 9, Temporary [Shampoo-Out] Color). A rinse can amplify your gray and make it look like shining, lustrous silk.

Now let me make a point about gray hair you may not have known. *Dryness.* Gray hair tends to be the driest of all hair types. There's less moisture in gray hair, so to keep it looking soft and bouncy, remoisturizing becomes very important. Regular deep-conditioning treatments are something I recommend to every gray-haired client I have.

And there's *another* very important point about gray hair I want you to be aware of: Gray hair tends to be *straighter* than hair with natural pigment. Even if you have had wavy or curly hair all your life, once you are totally gray, you'll have a lot less natural wave to your hair. That's why so many women with gray hair have permanents regularly, to reestablish the waves or curls. But this can develop into a vicious cycle. Gray hair starts out fairly dry. Put a perm on top of that, and you lose even more moisture. Ladies, please, if you love your gray hair and have perms regularly, *lavish* conditioner on your hair often to keep it looking its shining, glossy best. Look at Barbara's Before picture again and you'll see her hair looks a bit fuzzy. That's because it was dry. Now look at her After photo once more. That's the way gray hair looks when it's been properly conditioned. Be sure *your* gray has the luster and glow of natural pearls.

In restyling Barbara's hair, we redesigned the cut to maximize the amount of fullness at the top. More height adds drama to her looks and carries the beauty focus to the top of her face and her eyes. In general, it's a good idea at this age to have an upward emphasis in any style you choose. It's simply prettier and makes the most of what you have. If you need to visualize the opposite for purposes of contrast, think of long hair hanging over the shoulders of a teenager. A sixteen-year-old face may be able to take that "downward mobility" but it's not a flattering direction for a face nearing sixty. "Onward and upward" is more like it!

Makeup for Barbara included soft, smoky eye shadow, liquid eyeliner in a deep taupe for definition, and a sliver of highlighting under the eyebrow to give her eyes a more open look. We penciled her eyebrows into a slightly higher arch, again to keep her looks going upward. Delicate cheek color and a soft raspberry-colored lipstick finished Barbara's makeup make-over.

Barbara's all set now and I'm glad I caught her when I did. Since we worked together, she's started *another* new life! A few months ago her husband was promoted and asked to relocate to his company's home office in Cincinnati. Did

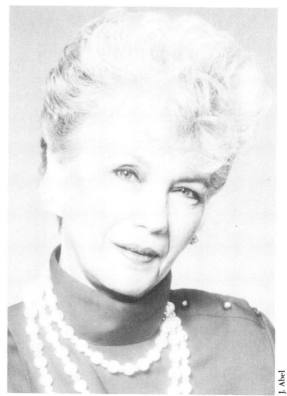

AFTER

J. Abel

Barbara have any qualms about packing bag and baggage and moving to the Midwest? Not her! Last time we talked, she was looking for a new house in Ohio. I'm sure this will be a great move for the Levees. Onward and Upward could well be their motto since it seems to describe to a T how they are planning to live the good life.

Lola Fisher

Age 58
Los Angeles, California
Actress, singer, college student
"This is wonderful. It's my
personal best."

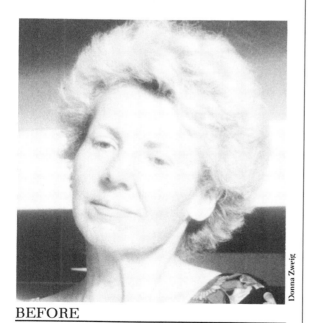

BEFORE

Donna Zweig

Working with Lola Fisher was a case of
"new beginnings" coming full circle—
for both of us. The last time I did Lola's
hair was over twenty-five years ago! She
was understudying the lead role of Eliza
Doolittle in *My Fair Lady* on Broadway
and her own hair had to be made a little
lighter to match Julie Andrews's, just in
case Lola had to go on. Then Sally Ann
Howes took over the lead role, and Lola
had to go *really* blonde. But the shade
suited her at the time and worked well,
both in Lola's personal and professional
life.

When Lola walked into the studio in
California where I was doing make-overs
for the "A.M. Los Angeles" television
show, we hugged each other long and
hard. It was a heartwarming reunion. A
lot of water has flowed under the bridge
since we last met. In the intervening
years, Lola had moved West and had
been pursuing her career there ever
since. She'd been married and then divorced. That experience had been very
emotional for her and had required a big
adjustment, but now Lola was back
working and in the process of relaunch-
ing her career. This time round, she is
going for the "young grandmother"
roles.

Lola felt she needed a "lift" for her
own sense of well-being and thought
some hair and makeup refocusing might
be just the ticket. I was delighted to see
her and thrilled to be able to help.
What's more, I could see that Lola's evaluation of her own looks was absolutely
accurate. She still looked wonderful, but

everything about her was looking a little faded and a little washed out. Lola has lots of natural energy, which is a blessing considering her business. When auditioning for a role, that energy has to show right away. The minute she picks up a script she has to be "on." Lola's a real pro and while her wonderful energy often carries the day for her, I felt it wasn't coming through as quickly as it could in her looks.

I understood why she was wearing so little makeup. When Lola *is* working, she wears so much of it that, between jobs, she likes to give her skin a rest and just moisturizes it like mad. But even allowing for the lack of makeup, I felt Lola needed more *color*. I wanted to give her a warm, Titian look, all siennas, peaches, and soft golden reds. While gray hair is fine for Barbara Levee, it wasn't working at all for Lola. She needed hair coloring to brighten her looks and put her back in the spotlight. To enrich her looks, she needed a hair-color shade that would put a real glow in her complexion.

Here's Lola looking bright, exciting, and full of pizzazz! "This is *wonderful*," she burst out when she saw herself on camera. "It's my personal best."

The shade I developed for Lola's permanent hair coloring was a light reddish blonde (see chapter 13, Leslie Blanchard's Favorite Salon Formulas). I liked the idea of slipping a little red into her blonde and thought I was being very creative until she told me that several mem-

bers of her family had red hair. We agreed my choice at least had been intuitive! And oh, what a difference it made in warming up her complexion. We've talked about skin getting paler with age and the need to restore some of that lost warmth with hair color, but here you can *really* see how beautifully the spillover effect from her warm hair color enlivens her skin. Even without makeup, her hair will keep her looks warm, sunny, and vibrant.

Lola has fabulously thick hair that is a terrific asset, but she has to be ruthless about getting it trimmed regularly, otherwise it starts weighing down her looks. That's what had happened in her Before picture. But the minute we cut Lola's hair and released the natural bounce, her hair was able to hold its new style beautifully. Again, fullness is concentrated at the top to draw the eye up, to make Lola seem taller, and to focus attention on her eyes and cheekbones.

"Fresh" is the word I like to use when describing how a woman this age should look. That's the approach we used for Lola's makeup, too. This effect is achieved through less dependence on color than on *definition*. Eye shadow is a gray-blue shade to frame her eyes. Foundation is creamy beige for smoothing the skin tone, and blusher is a sheer apricot. Lipstick is a peachy tan and looks perfect with Lola's new, warm appearance. And of course, the eyeliner is very important. As the tissue around the eyes "relaxes" with the years, eyeliner can emphasize your eye shape beautifully. It also can

Jan Kennedy

Age 28
Fullerton, California
Wife, mother, actress

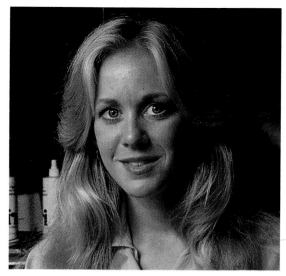

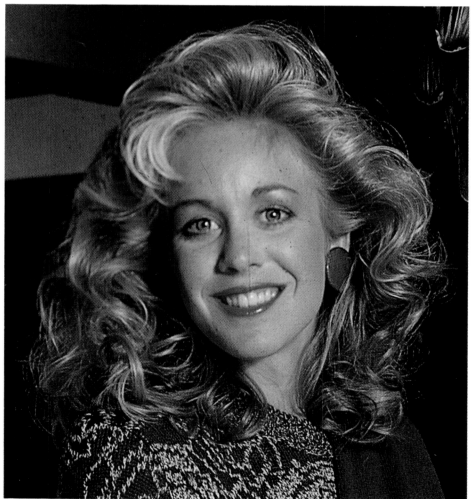

"I have a new, more exciting view of myself."

Photographs by Donna Zweig

Karen Risi

Age 29
Jackson Heights, New York
Import expediter

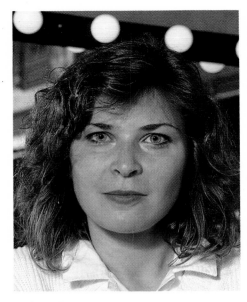

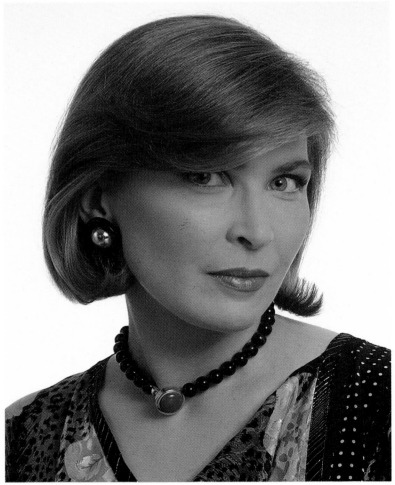

"A polished image counts in my business."

:Photographs by Donna Zweig

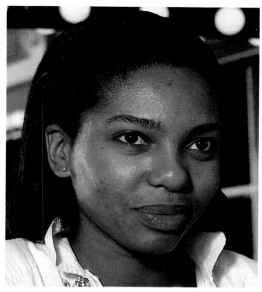

Stephanie Tucker

Age 25
Seattle, Washington
Model/actress

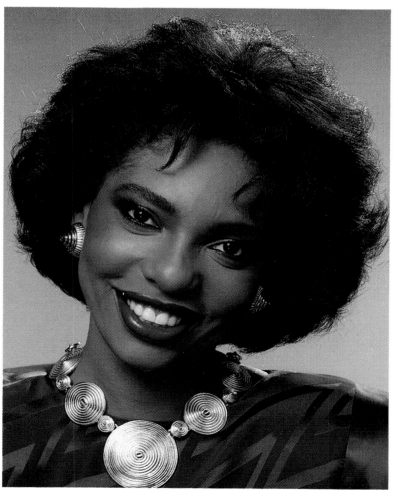

"Sophistication suits me fine…I love it."

Photographs by Donna Zweig

Kim Hankin

Age 31
New York, New York
Commercial real estate broker

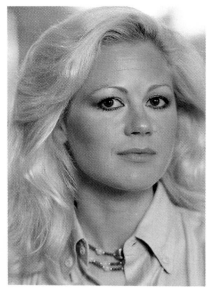

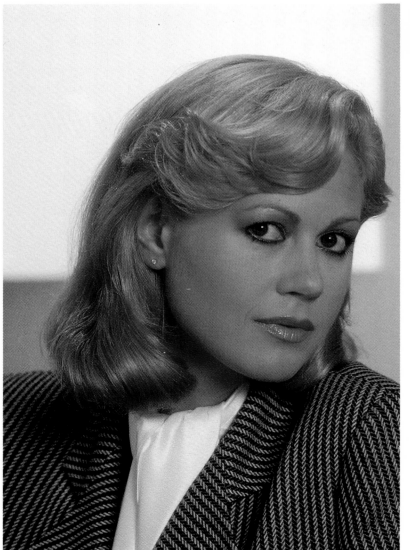

*"I look more like myself now,
and much more professional."*

Photographs by J. Abel

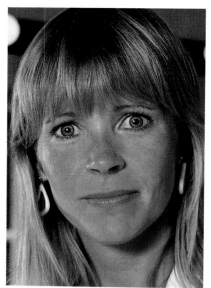

Gail Kislevitz

Age 34
Ridgewood, New Jersey
Wife, mother, consultant

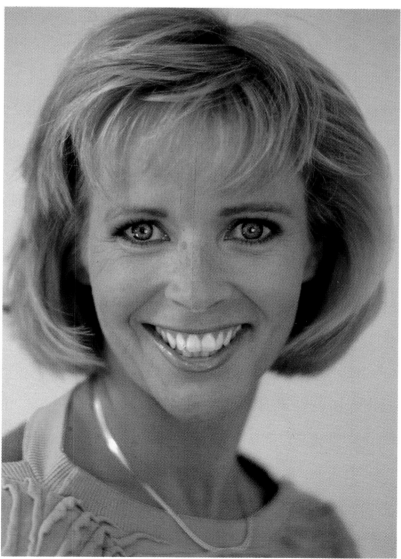

"This is the best I've ever looked!"

Photographs by Donna Zweig

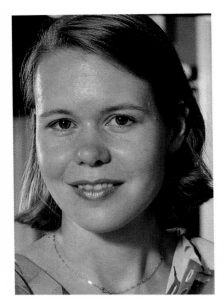

Sandy Thompson

Age 35
New York, New York
Graphic designer

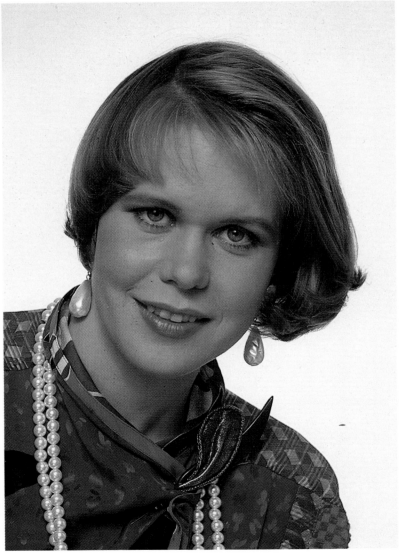

"My looks really fit me now."

Photographs by Donna Zweig

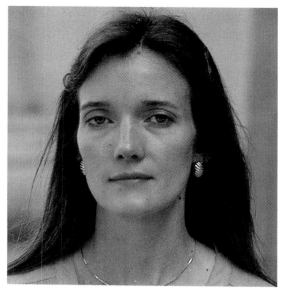

Patricia Bloom, M.D.

Age 35
Hastings-on-Hudson, New York
Wife, mother, physician

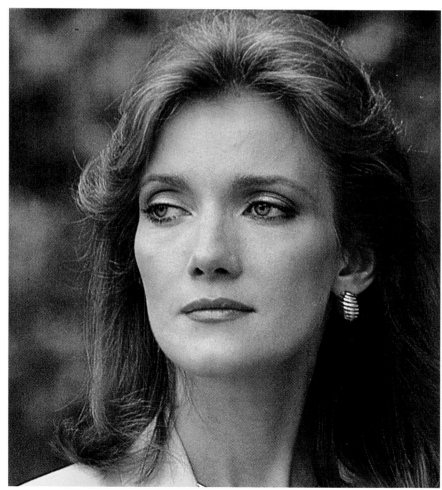

"I'll never go back to wearing barrettes!"

Photographs by Donna Zweig

Melissa Thornton

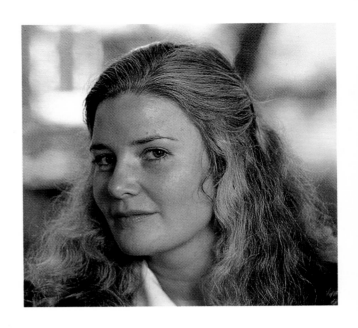

Age 33
Trumbull, Connecticut
Entrepreneur, real estate
developer

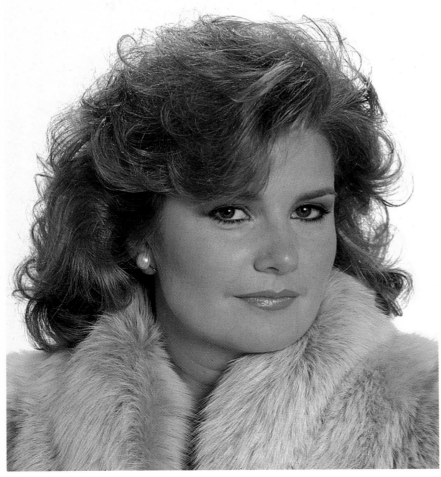

"I feel very, very elegant."

Photographs by J. Abel

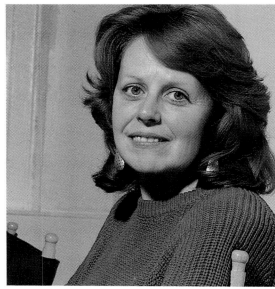

Barbara Aversano

Age 40
Lynbrook, New York
Sales administrator

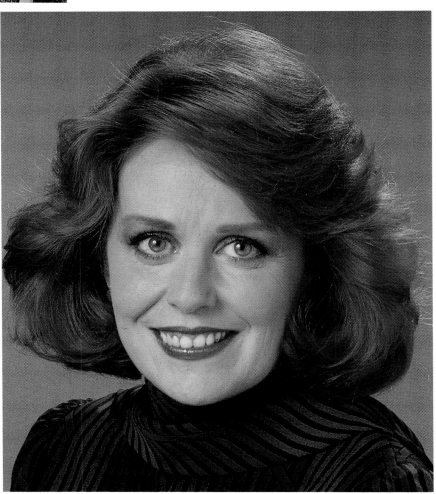

"*I'm* amazed *I can look this good.*"

Photographs by Rick Guidotti

Sandie McCarthy

Age 43
Cypress, California
Wife, mother, model,
community volunteer

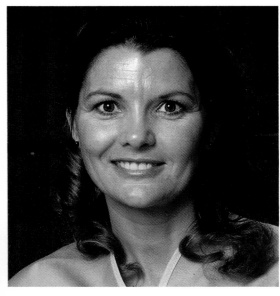

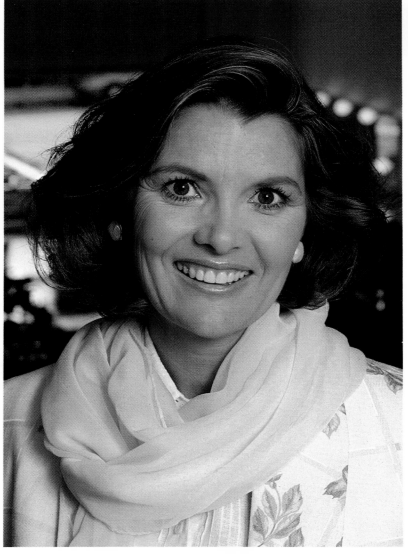

"I feel I've been set free!"

Photographs by Donna Zweig

Kay Bartlett

Age 45
New York, New York
Wire-service feature writer

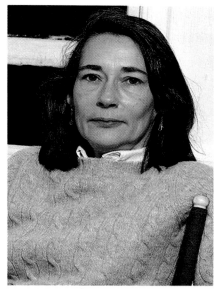

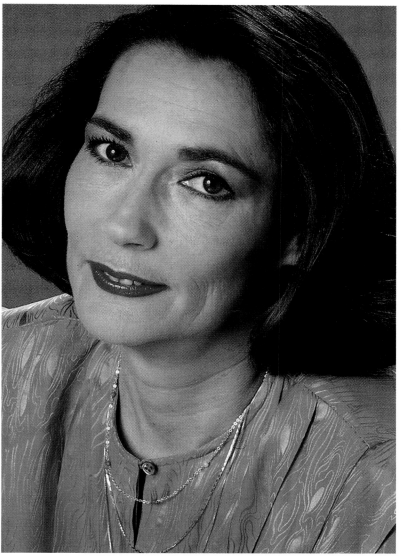

"I'd forgotten I could look this good."

Photographs by Rick Guidotti

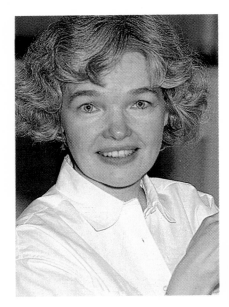

Karin Bardram

Age 49
Essex Fells, New Jersey
Wife, mother of four

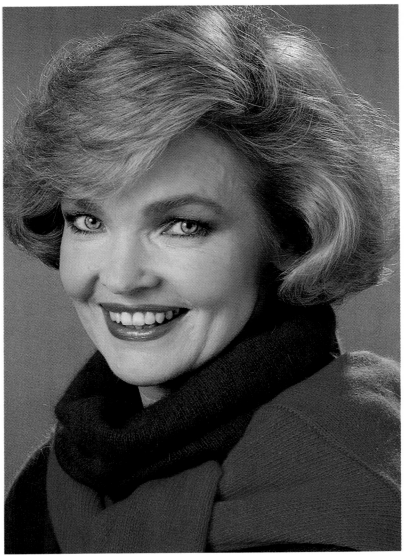

"I feel so much lighter!"

Photographs by Rick Guidotti

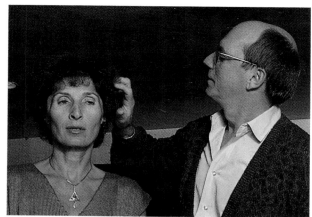

Rhoda Friedman

Age 48
Newport Beach, California
Wife, mother, community
volunteer

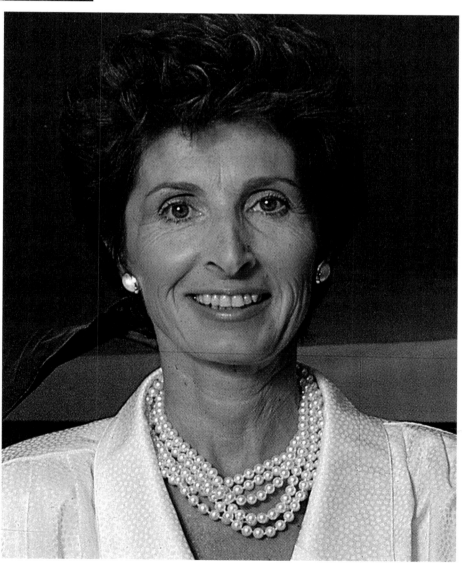

"I've never looked better."

Photographs by Donna Zweig

LaVonne DelCol

Age 51
Chappaqua, New York
Mother, assistant store manager

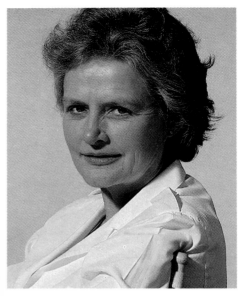

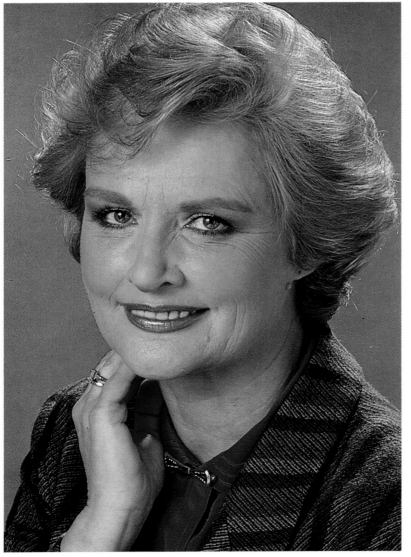

"Now I feel set for the next decade."

Photographs by Rick Guidotti

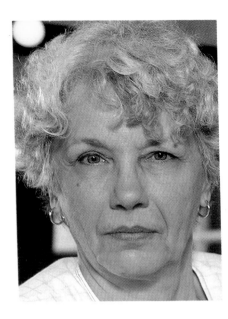

Barbara Levee

Age 56
Cincinnati, Ohio
Wife, mother, stepmother

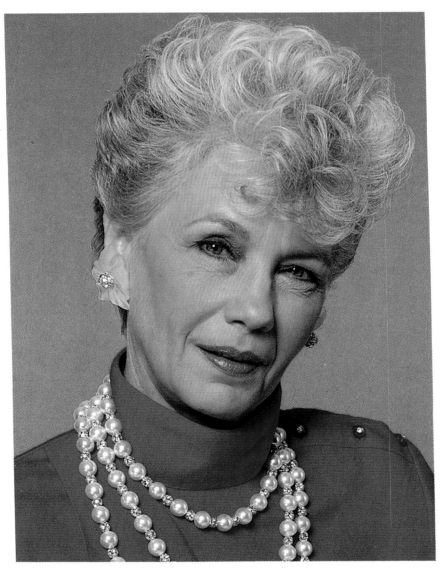

"This is the best style I've ever had in my life!"

Photographs by J. Abel

Lola Fisher

Age 58
Los Angeles, California
Actress, singer, college student

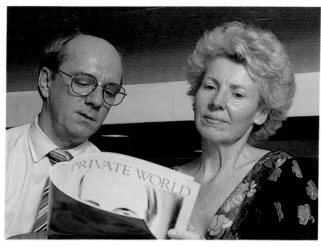

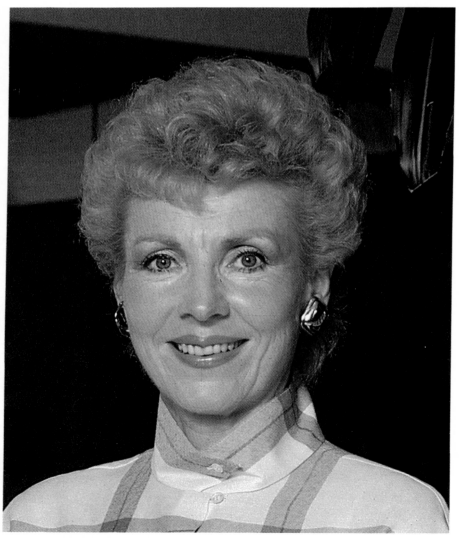

"This is wonderful. It's my personal best."

Photographs by Donna Zweig

make the whites of your eyes look whiter and brighter. I'm not suggesting a hard-edged look (*never* use black eyeliner unless you're onstage in full Grand Opera makeup), rather, a soft look that defines and brings out the dimension of your eyes. That's why we took particular care in choosing and applying the walnut-brown liquid eyeliner we used on Lola.

Once we were all finished, I looked at her and said, "Isn't life exciting? Here you are playing the mature part in the play and loving every minute of it." I really admire this woman. Because of her business, she can be working around the clock or have great chunks of time on her hands between jobs. But when she's not working, she uses her time very well. She's always wanted a college degree, so recently she went back to school and is studying for an Associate Arts degree. She's debating between concentrating her studies in child development or geriatric care (her own mother is in her nineties). Both fields appeal to her and both are challenging. She will take a few more courses before she decides.

Lola still auditions, still sings all the time (she's a lyric soprano), and is looking forward to getting her career re-launched successfully enough to spend time on both coasts. "After all, I spent the first third of my life in New York," she comments. She's also looking forward to a new relationship with a man she's yet to meet. That's great too. "And," she says, "I'm looking forward to never retiring. If an actress in her eighties can become a star doing a ham-

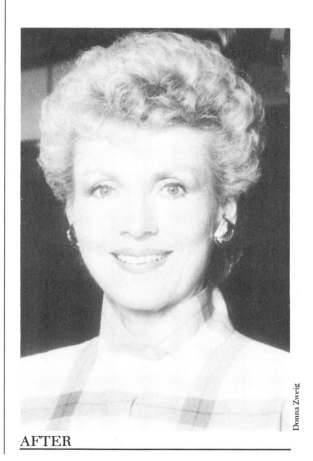

AFTER

Donna Zweig

burger commercial, think of how much is in store for me. I've got twenty years on her!"

Lola has lots of looking forward, but she's making the most of her life right now, too. It's a great time in her life or anyone else's. It's the perfect time to leave no stone unturned in trying *anything* you've ever been curious about trying. It's the time to s-t-r-e-t-c-h yourself, challenge yourself. You'll find the energy the minute you need it. You may have some talent that was always there just begging to be developed. Develop it now. Be one of the women who understands that the good life is as much about doing what you like doing as it is about learning how to do something new. And while you're in the process of discovering the real excitement of living the good life, I want you to *look* the best you've ever looked. Like Lola Fisher, I want you to be able to look in the mirror and say, "This is definitely *my* personal best!"

Part Two

APPLICATION

6

Hair-Coloring Methods

There are as many methods of coloring hair as there are women with different hair-coloring objectives, as you've seen in our make-overs. While enhancing the color of your hair always results in a wonderful change for the better in the way you look, a giant step is not always required to make that change happen. Sometimes a mere pointing up of your natural hair color is enough to work the magic. In other cases, however, particularly when your hair is very faded or very gray, the improvement in your looks can be so dramatic that it can make you feel like a whole new person.

On the pages that follow, I'll be taking you through all the different ways you can color your hair. We'll talk about preparing to color your hair, then help you pick the color that is perfect for you. From there, I'll discuss each hair-coloring method in detail. These chapters are arranged in order of *how much of a difference* each method can make in your looks—from a temporary rinse that washes out in the next shampoo, to frosting that lasts four months.

In order of how much change each coloring method can effect, we will discuss the following:

Temporary color that shampoos out right away
· Semipermanent color that washes off in four to six shampoos
· Highlighting
· Permanent color that stays put
· Overall frosting

With the coloring methods arranged this way, you can "plug in" at whatever level of change suits you best. If you are at all unsure, the foolproof and most conservative way to select a hair-coloring method is to start with temporary color, then progress through the subsequent methods, increasing the degree of color impact as you go. Some women begin coloring their hair with temporary color and, as they begin to go grayer and grayer, advance to the more dramatic methods, going full circle by the time they are completely gray and back to temporary color. That's one of the best reasons I can offer to encourage you to read through all the methods chapters at least once to give yourself an accurate idea of all the wonderful possibilities that await you.

7

How to Color Your Hair at Home

There has never been a better time to take hair coloring into your own hands. It's a smart, modern way to go about improving your looks. Further, the variety of products available, the improved formulations, the expanded number of shades, and the choice of methods currently on the market (temporary color to allover frosting) mean you can be sure of finding the hair color that's perfect for you.

Believe the Instructions

Home hair-coloring products are easy to use, safe, and will do everything they promise—providing you follow the instructions *to the letter*! Hundreds of thousands of dollars have been spent testing every single one of the products you see on the supermarket or drugstore shelf. The methods for using each of the products have been tried and tried again to work out every conceivable kink so you can do it yourself perfectly, even if it's your first time. The number of minutes you should leave the product on your hair has been tested over and over again. Every product has an automatic color "turnoff" and will not develop any further beyond the maximum number of minutes indicated. The most important thing you can do when using home hair-coloring products is to *believe the instructions*! Don't fall into the trap of reinterpreting the directions (what you think they *really* mean). Save your creativity for selecting the shade you want your hair to be.

Too Little Color

One of the most frequent mistakes I see women make is failing to leave a hair-coloring product on their hair for the full time specified in the instructions. They take one look in the mirror, panic, and wash everything off because they think that's the color their hair is going to be. Please listen to me. The color of the product as it is developing on the hair is normally *darker* than it will be when finished. That's the way it's *supposed* to look. Washing the color off too soon will result in only a pale approximation of what the color is designed to be. When covering gray (which can be particularly color-resistant), the pale approximation can result in pastel-tinted gray hair, not the full covering or highlighting you wanted. If that happens to you, don't blame the manufacturer. Go back, do it again, and this time leave the color on according to the directions (minus, of course, the number of minutes you had it on your hair the first time).

The Color Preview

Generally, to avoid any surprises in what shade your hair will be after coloring, I highly recommend the "strand test" or "color preview."

Here's how to do it:

1. Snip a lock of hair one-quarter inch wide at the roots. If you're brightening or lightening your hair, take a lock from the back at the nape where hair is naturally darkest. If you're covering gray, snip the lock from the grayest area—an inch back from the hairline at the temples, usually. Tape strand together at the roots.

2. Mix a small amount of the hair color you intend to use in a glass or plastic bowl and submerge the lock in the mixture.
3. Start timing. After twenty minutes, wipe the lock clean and check the color. If the hair isn't the color you want, return the lock to the mixture and let it absorb more color. Continue to wipe and check at five-minute intervals. What you're looking for is how long it takes the color to penetrate your hair. Leaving the lock in the mixture longer does *not* result in darker hair, but it does result in turning the hair the rich color you want it to be. However, if after a maximum of forty-five minutes the hair still isn't the color you anticipated, you may have to choose a different hair-color shade—lighter, brighter, or darker.

Another factor to consider in evaluating color is that when hair is wet (as the test strands will be), it looks darker than it will look when dry. If you're not completely sure of the shade by simply eyeing the lock of hair you are testing, rinse it off and hold it in front of a blow dryer for a few minutes. Then hold the dry lock of hair against your face and look in the mirror to check for depth of color.

Too Much Color

The first-time user of at-home hair coloring is the person apt to get too little color. The opposite problem—too much—happens to the woman who's been coloring her hair at home for a while and whose hair is suffering from color buildup. In this case, the hair coloring has been applied all over the head, time and time again, over a period of months and even years. The resulting color buildup makes hair look dull, usually too dark, and generally lifeless.

If you've already erred on the side of too much color, there are color "lifters" you can use at home. Once again, follow the directions very carefully. Or you can seek out the advice of a professional at a salon.

The Shampoo-in Error

A major misconception that I find among women who color their hair at home is this: If the color shampoos *in,* it must shampoo *out,* right? Wrong! The only type of color that shampoos out immediately is called "temporary" color and you will see the word "temporary" used both on the box and in the instructions. Otherwise, when the color shampoos in, you are using *either* semipermanent color, which stays in for four to six shampoos, or permanent color, which will have to grow out or be cut off if you want to get rid of it. Before buying a product because you like the description of the color, open the box and read all of the instructions. In particular, check the "retouch" segment. While shampooing the product into your hair may be fine the *first* few times you use it, look to see if root-area retouching is suggested thereafter. If that is the recommended method for ongoing maintenance, you can be sure that you are *not* buying a temporary or semipermanent hair-coloring product, whether or not it's a shampoo-in. If you're still unsure of which type of product you're buying, see chapter 10, Color That Gradually Wears Off (Semipermanent Color).

The Allergy or "Patch" Test

While the "strand" test to check color, described earlier, is one I highly recommend, the allergy or "patch" test is a *must.* The purpose of this test is to determine if you are overly sensitive or allergic to the hair-coloring product you plan to use. Just as some people are allergic to certain foods, cosmetics, or animals, others may be sensitive to the ingredients used in certain hair-coloring products. Also, our bodies go through different changes all the time. You may be taking a new medication, experiencing hormonal changes, or on a new diet. You even may be switching from one form of hair-coloring product to another. In all cases, it is imperative that you take the patch test each time you apply hair coloring.

Here's how it's done:

1. Mix a small amount of the coloring product in a small nonmetal dish (a saucer is fine). (You can use some of the mixture for a strand test at the same time if you like.)
2. Wash an area about the size of a quarter inside your elbow or behind one ear. Pat dry and apply a few drops of the color mixture.
3. Let the mixture dry, undisturbed and uncovered, for twenty-four hours. During that time do *not* put a plastic strip over the spot or, if you've applied the color inside your elbow, don't wear a tight-fitting, long-sleeved sweater.
4. If after twenty-four hours you see no adverse reaction, you can go ahead with your hair coloring. If, however, you notice any redness, swelling, burning, or itching of the skin, you have a hypersensitivity to the product and should not be using it.

In all my years as a professional, I have seen very few allergic reactions to the patch test. However, they can occur, so why take the chance? If, like the vast majority of women, you have no sign of irritation from the patch test, you can go right ahead and color your hair.

Final Preparations

The directions contained in any product box will tell you exactly what equipment you'll need to color your hair with that particular product. For the most part, these are ordinary items (towel, timer, glass, or plastic bowl). I have a few suggestions of my own, however, which I'd like to add.

If you are coloring your hair by yourself and will be using a root-application method, adding highlights all over your head, or if you're frosting your hair using a cap, I strongly recommend a two-mirror arrangement to give you a clear view of the back of your head while keeping your hands free to do the coloring. You can use a mirror that loops around your neck as you stand with your back to the bathroom mirror. Or use a wall-mounted mirror on accordion extensors that offers the same view. Being able to see the entire back of your head is very helpful in getting your roots or streaks done perfectly. An alternative to the two-mirror arrangement is to do your color with a friend. Each of you can help the other with the hard-to-reach areas.

Some women who regularly color their hair at home and know exactly what color is best for them buy two boxes of the product at a time. Keeping one box in reserve saves them another buying trip. When storing the extra product, however, do remember to keep it in a cool, dry place. And you must know that once you've combined the elements of any hair-coloring product into a mixture, you cannot save the remainder to use another time. You must discard any extra mixture immediately.

As for a timer, I prefer the type that has an audible bell that rings when the prescribed number of minutes has elapsed. I use the bell-ringer type of kitchen timer in my salon all the time. It lets us know exactly when time is up and color should be rinsed off. You'll find that the sound of a bell ringing saves you from having to remember if you started your timing five minutes before or after the hour.

Finally, I'd like to suggest you approach coloring your hair at home as a treat to yourself. Think of it as your own private time. Close the door. Tape a Do Not Disturb sign on it. Relax. Page through a fashion magazine or watch TV. If you want to call a friend for a chat, fine. Just be careful you don't color the earpiece of your white telephone in the process! And be alert for the sound of your bell timer. Enjoy these few minutes you're spending on yourself. Not only are you giving yourself a well-deserved break, you are going to look terrific when you're through!

8

Picking Your Perfect Hair Color

The single most important decision you'll be making in coloring your hair is, What shade should it be? What color will flatter you most? Will you look your best in hair that is lighter, darker, or brighter? What if you want to cover your gray?

In the next few pages, I'm going to take you through all the factors to consider when making a shade selection. This is the same way I develop color suggestions for my private clients. In this case, that client is you. I want you to understand everything that goes into making that all-important color choice. I cannot stress enough how important it is to explore all the color possibilities in full so you will be completely confident in making the color choice for yourself.

Warm or Cool

Let's start by determining if you are a "warm-" or "cool-" color person. As you look more closely at hair-color shades, you'll find there are cool blondes and warm blondes, cool browns and warm browns, cool brunettes and warm brunettes. There are even cool highlights and warm highlights. This very basic division between cool and warm colors first became apparent to me over twenty-five years ago and remains the first element I consider in determining what shade will suit you best. Cool colors are not flattering to a warm-color person and vice versa.

How can you tell if you are "cool" or "warm"? That distinction depends entirely on your complexion, so picking your best hair color starts with taking a close look at your skin. Hair and skin are the twin beauty basics and *must* work together if you are to look your best. What you want to do is determine if your particular complexion has a pink, cool cast or a golden, warm cast. All the decisions you make regarding your hair color will be based on this fact.

To tell if you are "cool" or "warm," take a very close look at your skin in *natural daylight.* Fluorescent light, because it is green, will make your skin look cool. Similarly, incandescent light bulbs give a yellow light and so make your skin look warm. I have northern light in my New York salon, which is the same light artists use, because it is the most accurate in which to evaluate color. So if you can, look at your skin in the ideal light, north daylight.

Do *not* use your face to judge your cool or warm complexion tone. The reason for this is that you may still have a little tan, which could throw your judgment off. Also, you may have a few burst capillaries that will make your skin look pink at first glance even though you really have golden warm skin. Similarly, if your skin tends to be sallow, your face may look golden, when in actuality yours is a cool complexion.

The best place on your body to examine your skin is inside your wrist or elbow. Now hold a piece of dead-white paper or a white tissue next to your skin. By comparison, does your complexion look pink with a blue undertone, or does it look golden with a yellow undertone? If you are unsure, compare your skin to another person's. Sometimes you can see your own skin tone more clearly that way, particularly if that other person's skin tone is different from yours. The other person could be a blood relative. All family members do not necessarily have the same skin tone. One brunette client of mine is a classic "cool." Her skin is very pink; this becomes dramatically apparent when you see her holding her three-year-old son, who is completely "warm," right down to his honey-blonde hair.

If you're still unsure if you are a cool- or warm-complexioned person (your skin color may be subtle), take a look at your wardrobe, your cosmetics, and your home. We sometimes *instinctively* pick colors that are right for us, colors we feel comfortable with, colors we know intuitively are flattering. Now ask yourself the following questions:

· When shopping for a light, neutral-colored sweater, do I gravitate toward pale gray or beige?
· In choosing a coat I can "wear over everything," would it be charcoal gray or chocolate brown?
· If I could own only one lipstick, would I be happier with peony pink or peachy coral?
· Redecorating my living room, which color scheme would "feel" better: taupe/cranberry/steel blue *or* camel/terra cotta/teal blue?
· Picking out wall-to-wall carpeting, would I opt for dove gray or cinnamon tan?

Choosing gray, peony pink, or taupe (the first color choices given in each question) means you are probably a cool-color person. The choices of beige, brown, coral, camel, or tan are warm-color-person choices.

Warm or Cool Hair-Color Shades

Now here's how to apply that "cool" or "warm" information to your hair-color choice. Every product you see will have a *shade name.* That particular name will tell you immediately if that shade is a cool color or a warm hair color. The tip-off words to look for if you are a "cool" are "ash," "moon," "smoke," and "blue." Tip-off words for "warm" are "beige," "sun," "gold," and "honey."

Do *not* trust the picture on the box! Hair-color manufacturers try their best to give you an idea of what the color inside really is, but there are too many vagaries in printing to have the true color come out accurately. The cardboard could be beige or gray, the ink pigments may be just that little bit off, the model may have that exact hair-color shade but the shiny paper on the carton makes it look lighter than it really is, and so forth. Also, differently named hair-color shades may look very similar in photographs, but have drastically different results when applied to your hair. For example, in photos Light Ash Blonde and Light Beige Blonde will appear to be almost identical. But once on your hair, Light Ash Blonde will look very cool, even silvery, while Light Beige Blonde will appear as a pale, golden blonde. To avoid making a mistake, always pick your hair color by its *shade name*!

To give you a very clear idea of how hair-color shades divide between being cool or warm, here is a table of common shade names used by major manufacturers (Clairol, L'Oreal, etc.):

COOL/WARM HAIR COLORING SHADE NAMES

Cool		Warm
Extra Light Ash Blonde Light Ash Blonde Moonbeam Blonde Medium Ash Blonde Dark Ash Blonde	—BLONDES—	Extra Light Beige Blonde Light Beige Blonde Sunbeam Blonde Strawberry Blonde Honey Blonde Dark Golden Blonde Reddish Blonde
	—REDHEADS—	Bright Copper Lightest Auburn Medium Auburn Dark Auburn Golden Brown Copper
Light Ash Brown Medium Ash Brown Moonlit Brown	—BROWNETTES—	Light Golden Brown Honey Brown Medium Golden Brown Sunlit Brown
Smoky Ash Brown Dark Ash Brown Darkest Brown Blue-Black	—BRUNETTES—	Dark Golden Brown Sable Brown Coffee Brown Brown-Black

Avoiding the Stereotypes

It is absolutely critical to choose either a cool hair-color shade or a warm one that will keep your skin and hair in perfect harmony. When evaluating your skin, however, do not fall into the trap of stereotyping yourself. For example, if you have a Celtic heritage, your may be trying to see the pink skin associated with that background. Don't forget that when the Vikings invaded Ireland and Great Britain in the tenth century, they left lots of golden-skinned blondes to mix in the generations that followed. Your family name may be Winchester, O'Brien, or MacGregor, but *you* may have the golden skin of a Scandinavian ancestor. And lest the blue-eyed blonde image associated with Denmark, Norway, and Sweden in itself become a stereotype, remember there are many "cool"-skinned brunettes from that part of the world. In other words, trust your eye, not your family name, when evaluating your complexion tone.

Ethnic Variations

Some variations on the cool/warm theme occur with Oriental skin. Nature has provided dramatic physical beauty for the Asian woman: golden skin set off by a crown of thick, dark hair. That natural combination is one I don't try to change in any substantial way. However, if an Oriental woman has very fair skin, I've found that shining up her black hair with a little warm brown gives the skin a wonderful glow. That warming of her hair color is, after all, completely compatible with golden skin. The cool shades, on the other hand, don't work well at all. I'd hate to see an Asian woman with ash-brown hair; it would make her skin look ashy, too.

One exception to the cool-warm rule pertains to the Oriental woman's makeup. She can look marvelous in either the warm or the cool cosmetic palette, and the *brighter* the better: vivid pink or socko-red lipstick, strong jade or teal eye shadow, intense pink or bright apricot blusher. She can suit her makeup to her wardrobe, which also should include some corresponding brights: carmine red, cobalt blue, magenta, vivid turquoise. Strong color looks wonderful on an Oriental woman, everywhere *but* her hair.

Black skin has its own variations, too. Because of the wide range of black skin tones, from very dark to very light, different guidelines are in order for different complexions. When it comes to hair color, I generally avoid "cool" colors, because, as with Orientals, ashy colors tend to make black skin look gray. The darker the skin, the less I depend on hair color to make a beauty impact, with the possible exceptions of a spray-on, "party" color for a festive evening. What I'm most concerned with is the condition of the hair itself. I want to see light, shine, and luster through the hair. Black hair is naturally fragile and if it has been "relaxed," it is all the more vulnerable to further damage. The most critical beauty action to take with dark black hair is to condition, condition, condition to keep it shiny and healthy looking.

At the medium and lighter end of the black skin spectrum, auburn and copper hair-color shades begin to look wonderful. There is a natural compatibility between medium to fair black skin and warm, vibrant hair color, particularly for the black woman with gold, hazel, or green eyes. But for all black women, nothing is as important as keeping your hair in healthy shape. If you are black and thinking about coloring your hair, please understand that your hair will look only as good as the condition it's in, so handle it carefully and give it regular deep-conditioning treatments to maintain its shine.

Makeup for black women runs the gamut of color possibilities. No one looks quite so wonderful as the dark black woman in cool cosmetic colors. What may not be right for her hair is perfect for her skin. The cool makeup shades that suit her include the entire pink-to-purple range. Dark black skin has an extraordinary affinity for all shades of rose, from deep to pale, for all the violets, from dark blue-violet to bright red-violet, and for all the wine colors from burgundy to rosé. I like the dark black woman to give a brilliant impression, but more in makeup and wardrobe than in hair color. For the medium to fair-skinned black woman, makeup in the "warm" cosmetic shades takes over. She looks great in terra cottas, corals, khaki greens, particularly if her hair is in the deep-auburn-to-copper hair-color range.

You can begin to see how important it is to understand how the cool and warm color palettes affect the choices you make in hair, makeup, and wardrobe. But what if you're just going gray? How does that work with the cool-or-warm rule?

Cool Gray and Warm Gray

Just as with all other hair-color shades, there are cool grays and warm grays. If you are a cool-color person, chances are your first gray hairs will grow in with a cool or blue cast. They can be very pretty and complement your pink skin. You may want to keep your gray, at least for a few years. By the time you're around forty-five, though, your gray hair may make you look older than you actually are. At that time, you may want to make another decision about your hair color.

If you are a warm-color person, your gray hair may come in looking yellow. Usually it is *not* a flattering look and in this case I advise the warm-color person to start covering the yellowish gray as soon as it has begun to become noticeable. There are several rich, vibrant shades the warm color person can choose from to complement her golden skin. Later in this chapter I will go into detail on covering gray, but I wanted you to realize now that even gray hair falls into the cool/warm categories, as do highlights.

Highlights and Frosting—Warm or Cool?

Just as gray hair can be either warm or cool, so can highlights and frosting. Highlights are added to hair that has little gray and usually ends up in the warm category. The reason for this is that all hair lightens in predictable stages: first to red, then to orange, then to gold, all of which are warm colors. To get a cool effect, as with frosting, you lighten your hair, then add a color wash over the lightened strands, usually in a cool color. Later on I have entire chapters devoted to these techniques, but I wanted to mention this to you now to show you that the hair-color impression you'll make is going to be warm or cool even if you don't color every hair on your head!

Now that we've reviewed all the hair-coloring shade options in the cool and warm categories, let's find out if you're going to look your best in a hair color that is lighter, darker, or simply brighter than your natural shade.

Lighter, Darker, or Brighter?

What we're talking about here is the amount of contrast between your hair and face that will flatter you most, bring out your eye color, and/or highlight your complexion. There are some very sound guidelines to follow when deciding how light or how dark you should go with your hair color. The first one is this:

Avoid extremes. The darker or lighter you go, the more perfect your features and skin have to be.

Think about it. The greater the contrast between your hair and your face, the more beautiful the features, the more flawless the complexion have to be to carry it off. Let's discuss these extremes. The lightest of light hair colors is white blonde. In the tens of thousands of women I've worked with, I've rarely seen a woman able to wear that light a shade successfully. Even if you were white blonde as a child, nature has darkened your hair to a deeper blonde color by the time you reached your adult years. Consequently, white-blonde hair on a grown woman always looks to me like the hair has been pushed too far to be believable, and usually it has. The bleaching that is required for that light a shade invariably strips the hair of any natural highlights or springiness and leaves it stiff and strawlike. That's why when a client comes to me with white-blonde hair, the first thing I do is to put her on a schedule of deep-conditioning treatments to get the hair back into shape, then wait until the hair grows out enough to handle it without doing even more damage. Further, in my view white-blonde hair smacks of old movie-star images from the 1930s and 1940s. It just doesn't look right for women of the 1980s.

The opposite of the light hair-color extreme is blue-black, which looks just as artificial to me as white-blonde hair. Blue-black hair requires perfect features, perfect makeup, and perfect maintenance—every hair must be in place at all times. It is a very, very hard color to wear because it is so draining and aging to the skin. Snow White may have had raven-black hair, but as far as I'm concerned, I'd leave blue-black hair to teenage girls in fairy tales where it belongs.

Let's get on to all the other prettier and more flattering color options open to you.

If you are considering coloring your hair for the first time, or even if you're in the process of rethinking your current hair color, here's another excellent guideline: *Pick a hair-color shade no more than two shades lighter or one shade darker than your natural color.*

Since nature never goes that far wrong, one to two shades lighter or one shade darker may be all you need to perk up your beauty image. Also, lightening or darkening your hair is always best done in gradual stages rather than in one melodramatic swoop you may regret later. You can always inch a little lighter or darker once you establish the general range of your best hair-color shade.

Picking a Lighter or Darker Shade

So you can see exactly where you are now as well as the color grouping you'd be going into when selecting one or two shades lighter or one shade darker, here is a table showing the light-to-dark range of hair-coloring shades you can choose from. The actual shade names are the same ones listed in the cool/warm table, but this time I've assigned each shade a color value, starting with 1 for the lightest and ending with 11 for the darkest. Within each numbered level, the cool shades are listed first, then the warm shades.

Using This Chart

Say your natural hair color is medium brown (which most women call "mousy brown"). You would start out with the medium browns that are listed at level 7 on the chart. If you are a cool-color person, you could move up to Light Ash Brown on level 6 or, for maximum lightening, go for Dark Ash Blonde on level 5. For darkening, you would go down to level 8 with Smoky or Dark Ash Brown. If you are a warm-color person with medium-brown hair, you could lighten to Honey Brown on level 6 or go even lighter with Reddish Blonde on level 5. For a deeper, more dramatic color, you would choose a shade from level 8, Dark Golden Brown or Dark Auburn.

LIGHT-TO-DARK HAIR-COLOR SHADES

Shade Name	Level	Shade Name	Level
Extra Light Ash Blonde Extra Light Beige Blonde	1	Moonlit Brown Sunlit Brown Medium Ash Brown Medium Golden Brown Medium Auburn Golden Brown Copper	7
Light Ash Blonde Light Beige Blonde	2		
Moonbeam Blonde Sunbeam Blonde Strawberry Blonde	3	Smoky Ash Brown Dark Ash Brown Dark Golden Brown Dark Auburn	8
Medium Ash Blonde Honey Blonde	4		
Dark Ash Blonde Dark Golden Blonde Reddish Blonde Bright Copper	5	Coffee Brown Darkest Brown Sable Brown	9
Light Ash Brown Honey Brown Light Golden Brown Lightest Auburn	6	Brown-Black	10
		Blue-Black	11

As you see, I've included very light blondes (level 1) and blue-black (level 11) in this chart. The reason I've done so is to establish the extremes.

Also, *very* occasionally I may use half a capful of a very light or very dark color in a formula for extra drama, but never, *never* for an entire head of hair. Most women will find themselves very comfortable in the six color levels between 3 and 8.

We've talked about too much contrast between the hair and the face and why you should avoid the extremes. But the flip side of too much is having too *little* contrast. This occurs when a woman finds that her hair and skin tone blend together too closely, with the hair not providing enough of a frame for her features.

Too Little Contrast

One example of too little contrast is the pale-skinned "dishwater" blonde. Another is the redhead who has been out in the sun and finds her hair too light and her skin too dark. Still another example is the woman of Mediterranean or Hispanic background whose hair has faded (whether from age or the elements), so hair and skin together now just look "muddy." Too little contrast between hair and face, whether from genetics, age, or a seasonal change, is easily corrected. The same 1–2 up, 1 down rule applies. One or two shades lighter or one shade darker is all that is needed to refocus your looks and get your hair back into the shade range that offers the prettiest frame for your particular complexion and features.

Brightening Your Hair

You may not need to either lighten or darken your hair. If you are generally pleased with the contrast between your hair and skin, yet still feel you look a little "blah," brightening may be all you need. "Brightening" means you stay within your own color level, going neither darker nor lighter, just to a more interesting shade. This is the most conservative step you can take in changing the color of your hair. Brightening simply intensifies the natural color and energizes your hair's appearance by adding new sparkle and lots of shine.

Let's take the woman with the mousy-brown hair again. She could be an ideal subject for brightening. Within her own level she can dramatize her hair with Moonlit Brown if she's a cool-color person, or give her hair a real boost with Medium Auburn if she's a warm-color person. All you do when brightening is to stay within your own natural light-to-dark level, but pep up your existing color. Older women who don't have much gray are wonderful candidates for brightening. But whatever your age, if your hair looks dull to you when you look in the mirror, consider brightening things up a bit. You'll probably love the improvement!

So far we've discussed cool/warm colors plus how to choose a shade that is lighter, darker, or brighter. The third part of your color consultation has to do with covering gray.

Going Gray

Gray hair is *not* hair that has turned a different color. In fact, it has turned *no* color. What has happened is that the hair root stops producing natural color pigment. Thus, the hair strand no longer contains any blonde, brown, or red pigment. Ninety-nine and nine-tenths percent of gray hair is due to the normal aging process. The other one-tenth of one percent may be due to an acute vitamin deficiency, the type usually seen in Third World countries where famines regularly occur. As for hair turning gray "overnight," it just doesn't happen. The color a hair shaft will be on its surface begins deep within the hair root at the commencement of its growth. Thus, you may meet a friend you haven't seen for a while who looks as if he or she has suddenly turned gray, but if you think for a minute, you might not have seen that person face-to-face in over a year, the time it normally takes for a complete head of hair to grow in gray. And that's a speedy extreme.

Normally the graying process begins very subtly. Hair begins to get a little drab, fading a bit all over. A few gray hairs begin to appear at the front hairline around the forehead and the temples. Then a few more. Eventually, gray hairs are scattered throughout the drab and faded color, giving the hair a no-color look. This normal process of graying starts when we are in our late twenties and early thirties.

Percentages of Gray

It is helpful to learn how to describe amounts of gray hair in terms of percentages, which is the way hair professionals generally do it. I want you to think of your gray hair this way because there are several different coloring methods I advise, all depending on how gray your hair has become. As the amount of gray increases, the preferred hair-coloring method changes, too.

For example, the just-beginning-to-go-gray woman who has a few gray hairs around the edges of her hairline near her face would be considered five to ten percent gray. She's simply lost a little color, so all she has to do is to add some. This can be done with temporary rinses, color that gradually wears off, or any other method she likes.

Ten to twenty-five percent gray means that when you look in the mirror, you can see gray hair beginning to appear all over your head. It is not just concentrated at the temples and front hairline; rather, the gray is sprinkled throughout the hair. Because gray hair can be resistant to coverage, temporary color will not cover enough. For decent coverage, you will be best off using either semipermanent color (the type that gradually shampoos off) or permanent color.

Twenty-five to fifty percent gray is what you have if your hair no longer looks a definite color. The gray impression has built not only because of the number of gray hairs, but because your basic natural color has become quite drab. To cover twenty-five to fifty percent gray you may be able to use semipermanent color at the lower end of this range. In the upper ranges between thirty-five and fifty percent, permanent color will give you better coverage.

More than fifty percent gray means that anyone meeting you for the first time will describe you as gray-haired. That's the impression your hair gives. In general, the grayer you get, the more permanent the hair color you should use to cover the gray. And with over fifty percent gray, permanent color is the only realistic choice you should consider if you want to cover the gray.

More information on each of the coloring methods follows, each in its own chapter (chapters 9 through 12), but it's appropriate that you fix in your mind how much gray hair you have now so you can make an informed decision for the future.

Is Gray Hair Different?

You bet it is! First, at the same time that the hair root has stopped producing its pigment, it has also reduced the amount of oil and elasticity normally contained in the hair shaft. Thus, gray hair can be wiry and difficult to handle. That's why some women find that their gray hairs stick out more than the hair that still contains natural pigment. Conditioning helps, and for some women is an absolute necessity.

Second, because gray hair is generally coarser, it may resist hair-color application. Therefore, it is mandatory to keep whatever coloring product you use on your hair for the fullest time suggested, if you want the color to penetrate the hair shaft and give you full coverage.

Coloring Over Gray Hair

The most significant difference between gray hair and naturally pigmented hair becomes apparent when you apply color. Think of it as if you were painting a wall. Any color you use on a white wall is going to appear clearly and immediately. If the wall you are painting is already a medium beige, the color you use on top is going to be modified in its clarity. Coloring your hair works on the same principle. Color applied over white-gray strands is going to be lighter and more noticeable than color applied on top of another color. Do *not* think of this as always being negative! Here's why: Hair is usually lighter in front, around the face, then slightly darker toward the crown, and darkest at the back of the nape where the sun never reaches it. Most often this is the same way hair goes gray. Consequently, when you apply color over gray, as a rule the new color will appear lighter around the face, gradually darkening toward the back. In effect, your own gray works as a very flattering highlighting system!

For example, if you apply Honey Brown coloring to medium drab brown hair with fifteen percent gray, most of the hair (the eighty-five percent that retains some pigment) will come up looking a rich, golden brown. On the fifteen percent of your hair that is gray, Honey Brown becomes a *light* brown with golden "highlights," giving your hair color dimension and a very pretty play of light through the hair.

As we've said, the color shade you choose will look just a bit lighter applied to gray hair. This is not as tricky as it sounds because of the highlighting effect just described. But I don't want you to be surprised when coloring your gray hair at home, so here's another chart showing what various hair color shades look like when applied to gray hair. To avoid any confusion, I'm using the exact same shade names used on the two previous charts so you can keep track of your own preferred shade.

HAIR-COLOR SHADES FOR COVERING GRAY

Name of Shade	Final Shade on Gray Hair
Extra Light Ash Blonde	Lightest cool blonde
Extra Light Beige Blonde	Lightest vanilla blonde
Light Ash Blonde	Light ash blonde
Light Beige Blonde	Light pastel blonde
Moonbeam Blonde	Light cool blonde
Sunbeam Blonde	Light warm blonde
Strawberry Blonde	Light strawberry blonde
Medium Ash Blonde	Light ash blonde
Honey Blonde	Light honey blonde

HAIR-COLOR SHADES FOR COVERING GRAY

Name of Shade	Final Shade on Gray Hair
Dark Ash Blonde	Medium ash blonde
Dark Golden Blonde	Medium warm blonde
Reddish Blonde	Light reddish blonde
Bright Copper	Bright red
Light Ash Brown	Dark ash *blonde*
Honey Brown	Light warm brown
Light Golden Brown	Light warm brown
Lightest Auburn	Very light auburn
Moonlit Brown	Light ash brown
Sunlit Brown	Light warm brown
Medium Ash Brown	Light-medium cool brown
Medium Golden Brown	Light-medium warm brown
Medium Auburn	Light auburn
Golden Brown Copper	Light reddish brown
Smoky Ash Brown	Medium ash brown
Dark Ash Brown	Medium ash brown
Dark Golden Brown	Medium warm brown
Dark Auburn	Medium auburn
Coffee Brown	Medium brown
Darkest Brown	Medium brown
Sable Brown	Medium brown
Brown-Black	Darkest brown
Blue-Black	Blue-black

Complexion Notes for Gray Hair

Just as the natural aging process causes hair to lose its pigment, the same effect occurs with the skin. As we grow older, the skin generates and retains less pigment. This makes the complexion look paler and a little gray, too.

For my clients with more than fifty percent gray (which I can see when I'm retouching their roots if they are already coloring their hair), two out of every three look best in a warm-hair-color formula to lend their complexions a little more of a glow. Even for my clients who are cool-color persons, I frequently include a few capfuls or so of a warm hair color to enliven their looks. If you are a older woman with over fifty percent gray, you may want to buy one home hair-coloring product for your major color, then buy a second shade for a bit more warmth (See chapter 13, Leslie Blanchard's Favorite Salon Formulas, for more details.)

Of course, judicious use of makeup helps the skin tone enormously. A light skimming of powder blusher all over the face is one way to do it. Or you can use a few dots of a liquid color product. Just be sure to blend well. And there is no question that regular exercise brings more natural color to the skin of a woman of *any* age.

Realistic Color Choices to Cover Gray

If you had glorious, deep chestnut-brown hair when you were a teenager, I have some bad news: You *cannot* go back to that deep a shade and still look good today. The reason is that trying to replicate the color of your youth is not only too difficult technically (did it have gold or auburn high-lights, for example?), but it is going to look too harsh on an adult woman's face, character lines and all. Also, choosing a dark color to use over hair that is gray or in the process of graying can make the hair look thinner than it is. Your best move is to aim for a color one shade or level *lighter* than your hair was when you liked it best. Thus, if you had dark-brown hair in your teens, go for a medium brown now. If you had medium-brown hair then, use a light brown now, and so forth. You'll be much more comfortable with the results and as long as you are somewhere in your natural hair-color range, your color will look more believable and much, much more flatter-ing.

Now that you know everything you need to know about picking your own perfect hair-coloring shade, I'd like to talk about the different ways you can color your hair. Frequently, the shade you've chosen will be avail-able in several coloring methods. If we use Honey Brown again as an example, you will find that shade in a hair-coloring product you rinse out every time you shampoo, one that will stay on your hair through five or six shampoos, and one that colors your hair permanently (meaning the color will stay put until it grows out or you cut it off). In the following chapters I will discuss each of these methods in detail.

Each method has its own advantages, so let me suggest you read through all of them, see if you identify with the statements that precede each chapter, and generally inform yourself thoroughly before making your choice.

9

Temporary (Shampoo-Out) Color

Can you identify with any of these statements?

"I've always had a hankering to see what I'd look like as a smoldering brunette."

"I'm going to a special party next weekend. I have a terrific dress, and some outrageous makeup. I want to dress up my hair, too."

"I've seen those first few gray hairs around my face, but have no idea what color I want to use. A brighter version of my own color may be enough for now."

"I'm due for a touch-up, but my hair is looking particularly brassy and I'd like to tone it down a little."

"My hair is completely gray and while I like it well enough, it gets boring. Maybe a little color rinse would help."

All of the above are good reasons to try temporary color, whether in the form of wild color streaks for a special evening or a quiet enhancement of your own natural color. All temporary products are designed to be used for the short term: As soon as you shampoo, out they go. While on the hair, however, temporary products make your hair more colorful as well as add body and some extra shine. But what is so appealing about this type of color is its very temporariness.

The Temporary-Color Explosion

New color excitement in temporary color is due to the dramatic expansion in the number of shades now available, plus the variety of great new ways you can apply that color. Good old liquid rinses are still with us, but in more colors than ever. Then there are all the terrific color mousses. Much like styling mousses you would finger-comb through your hair, these temporary color foams let you place color anywhere you like it. Want a little extra color at the temples? Concentrate your color mousse there. Want to try a new color all over your head? Help yourself. In addition, there are spray-ons for "hot stuff" streaks and bright gels in either a tube or a jar that you use like finger paints. The colors are riotous: hot pink, electric blue, neon green, cinnamon red, plum, bright gold, or tinsel silver. Think of them for fun and fantasy and for a fabulous evening.

Then there are all the temporary colors more closely related to real hair shades, but with a little extra zip. They give you an opportunity to spark up your color any time you like.

Temporary Color and Your Fashion Image

Say you've had light hair all your life and always wondered how you'd look as a redhead or with hair the color of black opals. Try it! The great part about using this type of color is that it lets you create dramatic surprises for yourself and others. With temporary color, you can treat your hair like a versatile fashion accessory. Just as you switch your makeup shades for certain outfits, you can consider temporary color as the new cosmetic for your hair. Say you just bought an aubergine jacket. Try a little Blueberry Mousse in your hair. A new biscuit-colored sweater? Some Spiced Cognac temporary color would look pretty. The wonderful part about these new temporary shades is that they're on your hair today and gone tomorrow. They give you a quick and easy way to change your hair color without any commitment to any particular shade. They're fast, fun to use, and a great way to play with different colors. You can be outrageous one day, low-key the next. These colors permit you to express yourself whatever mood you're in . . . or want to be in.

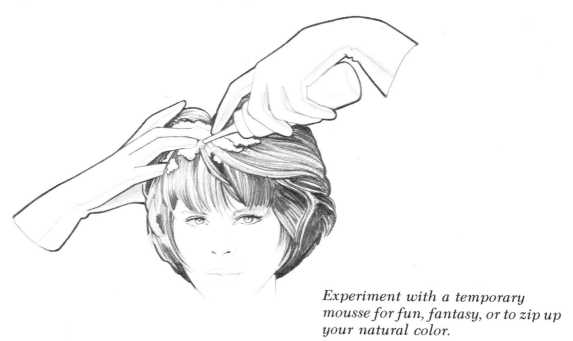

Experiment with a temporary mousse for fun, fantasy, or to zip up your natural color.

Enhancing Your Natural Color

Besides all the fashion statements you can make, there are some down-to-earth uses for temporary color, too. It's a wonderful way to enrich your natural hair color, for example, to show it off in its very best light. If you are a warm brown to begin with, some chestnut temporary color will give your hair extra glints of gold. Of if you're a cool brown, temporary color can pick out smoky highlights in your hair. Although the amount of change when using temporary color is not that great when close to your own shade, your natural color will nonetheless look more intense, more definite, and have extra glow and depth.

Temporary Color Auditions

Because temporary color washes out immediately, it's a perfect way to audition a color you're thinking of using. Many women try on temporary color when they first notice the odd gray hair making its appearance. While this type of color doesn't really cover gray, it does give you an idea of what a shade will look like on you. A liquid rinse will indicate how a warm or cool shade will look; a temporary mousse will give you an even better color audition. In using temporary color for this purpose, however, consider the color as a preview. If you like what you see, you can then opt for the full treatment. If, on the other hand, you feel a particular shade isn't quite right, you can go on to try as many others as you like. Since each will wash out in the very next shampoo, there's no harm being done to the hair as you experiment with different shades. You can keep trying as many colors as you like until you're completely comfortable with your choice.

Toning Down Brassy-Looking Color

If your hair color starts to look brassy, you may be using the wrong shampoo or not conditioning with one of the newer products that contain sunscreens. I suggest you read through the chapter on caring for your color-treated hair to learn how to avoid this happening in future. But for now, let's look at temporary color as a way of toning down brassiness on already tinted hair. It will work very well this way. If your color has gone "off," temporary color *will* refresh your color but only on a short-term basis. I suggest this only for the last shampoo or two before having your color retouched.

If you find your color becomes too brassy too soon and too often, however, you may have to rethink your color shade entirely. Is it too light to begin with? Would you be better off with one shade darker that would continue looking good retouch to retouch? Using a temporary rinse on color-treated hair is fine once in a while: when your regular hair color hasn't quite made it through a vacation in the sun, or you're a week to ten days past your regular retouch. Temporary color can be considered a great emergency method in those cases but should *not* be depended upon day in and day out.

Temporary Color on One Hundred Percent Gray Hair

When temporary color is used on completely gray hair, it can enhance your hair, but is always best in the lightest, most delicate tints. Sometimes all you may want to do is to make your gray sparkle, and temporary color will do that nicely. In other cases, a very little touch of color can do a lot to enliven your looks by complementing your complexion and eye color. But do *keep it light.* You've seen the mistakes, and heaven knows I have: the older woman with pink "cotton candy" hair or, even worse, the lady who looks like she used laundry bluing on her hair. The lightest vanilla, a touch of honey, a hint of moonlit platinum is plenty. Then again, if you have one hundred percent gray hair but also have the wardrobe, the face, the figure, and the verve, go for one of the temporary color mousses in an adventure-some shade like "red dazzle" that suits your energy and enthusiasm.

Regular Use of Temporary Color

If you find you really like using temporary hair color and that's as far as you ever want to go, great! However, if you use it every time you shampoo, be sure that every month to six weeks (or every eight to ten applications) you apply a heavy-duty conditioner to your hair and leave it on for fifteen or twenty minutes, or according to directions. Although you are washing the temporary color out of your hair with each shampoo, there may be just that tiny bit left in the hair, and this residue can build up over the weeks, dulling the shine in the process. A heavy-duty conditioner will not only leave your hair looking lustrous and shiny, it will help lift off any superfluous color that may have accumulated along the way.

One other fact for the regular temporary color user: If your hair has been relaxed or permed, wait a few days before applying any color. Hair is particularly porous right after being curled or straightened and may grab a little too much of the color pigment, even with temporary color. Wait until the *second* shampoo after perming or relaxing to use your temporary rinse, spray, gel, or mousse, and use less of the color the first time round.

TEMPORARY HAIR-COLOR ADVANTAGES:
- Offers dramatic hair color change you *don't* have to live with.
- Becomes a cosmetic for your hair and lets you use it as the newest fashion accessory.
- Let's you sport "sizzle" streaks for just one night.
- Is fun, fast, and easy to use.
- In quieter colors, enhances your natural shade.
- Permits you to "audition" a new hair color.
- Tones down brassiness as a short-term solution.
- Gives one hundred percent gray a beautiful, delicate hue flattering to skin and eyes.

TEMPORARY HAIR-COLOR LIMITATIONS:
- Will not completely cover gray.
- Will not compensate for an incorrect color choice in the long term.
- May run if you are caught in the rain.

10
Color That Gradually Wears Off (Semipermanent Color)

Are any of these statements true for you?

"I'm a hair-color beginner, but whatever I use, I don't want to be locked into touch-ups."

"I like my natural color but would like to see it without the gray that's beginning to show around my face."

"I'm not interested in lightening my hair, but I'd love to see it brighter and more dramatic, with more of a fashion image."

Because it is so easy to use, semipermanent color is a very popular method for both women *and* men, and there are many good reasons for its popularity. Semipermanent hair coloring is a wonderful introduction to hair color in general. Also, it's the perfect method to use for covering those first few strands of gray that may be diluting the natural color of your hair. In addition, it imparts a stronger color image to the hair, giving it a warmer touch of gold, or cooling it down to a smoky hue. Because of its ability to accent the prettiest positives in anyone's natural hair color, I consider semipermanent color the beginner's best friend. You almost can't make a mistake with it, so you can be fearless in your first color forays. What's more, it will pep up faded or dull hair, as well as giving the hair new gloss and a healthy shine.

Semipermanent color bridges the gap between temporary color that washes out the minute you shampoo your hair and permanent color that stays put until it grows out or is trimmed off. Semipermanent color shares a great advantage with temporary color, however: It requires *no retouching*. The color gradually wears off with each shampoo until it's time to refresh the color; then you reapply.

If you think of semipermanent color as "staining" the hair, you'll get the idea of what it does. This type of color does not penetrate very deeply, so the more often you shampoo, the faster it will wear off. My grandmother used to dip her white cotton gloves in hot tea to give them an "ecru" stain. After the gloves had been washed a few times, she would redip them to refresh the tint. Semipermanent color has the same effect on the hair and, after several shampoos, needs the same type of color refreshment to keep it looking bright and lively.

Semipermanent versus Permanent Color

As glorious as semipermanent color can be, do understand that it is a color "enhancer" and not your best choice for dramatic color change. While it adds rich, exciting depth to your own color, *semipermanent color will not lighten your hair.*

If you're looking for an allover lighter shade, you'll have to go to permanent color, which I will discuss in the next chapter. For now, let's take a closer look at semipermanent color. This is the one that *adds color* to what you already have. It does not contain any peroxide or "developer." In fact, some semipermanent hair-color products say No Peroxide on their boxes to emphasize the fact that they are not "lightening" products; they are covering and *enriching* products.

To distinguish semipermanent from permanent coloring products when shopping for your new hair color, look for phrases like "washes out gradually" or "up to 6 shampoos." Also, check to see if there is only one element in the box. If there are *two* elements in the package, one of which says Developer and you are supposed to *mix* the two elements together, you are handling *permanent* color, which does *not* "wash out gradually." Permanent color stays put until it grows out or you trim it off! Semipermanent color, on the other hand, requires *no mixing!*

The Great Shampoo-in Misconception

If you're still unsure whether you're looking at semipermanent or permanent hair coloring, here's another surefire tip: Look at the instructions for *retouching. Both* semipermanent and permanent color are applied for the first time using the shampoo-in method. But while semipermanent color *continues* to be applied that way, permanent color can also be retouched using the *root* retouch method. If instructions for how to apply color to the roots are included, I guarantee that you are handling a *permanent* color product. There is a significant difference between the two. If all you want to do is brighten your color or cover some gray, permanent color is more than you need.

If you remember nothing else in this book, please learn this statement by heart: *All shampoo-in hair color does not shampoo out.*

I cannot stress this point strongly enough. To name popular brand names, Clairol's "Loving Care" and L'Oreal's "Avantage" are both semipermanent hair coloring products that gradually shampoo out. If you are using Clairol's "Nice 'n Easy" or L'Oreal's "Preference," you are using *permanent* color that may shampoo in, but I guarantee it will *not* shampoo out. It's there to stay until it grows out or you cut it off.

Assuming that if you shampoo color *in* that it will shampoo *out* is the single most common misconception women have in using home hair-coloring products. The confusion is understandable, but I just don't want you to make that mistake and end up with more color than you bargained for. So when you're shopping for your semipermanent hair color, remember to look for only *one* product in the box you buy and only *one* suggested method of retouching (shampooing in). That will ensure you are buying semipermanent color.

Semipermanent Coloring Technique Tips

Many women use shampoo-in semipermanent hair coloring right after regular shampooing. That's fine, but not on soaking wet hair. The water retained in the hair will simply dilute the coloring product and give you less coverage than you want. Follow directions that call for towel drying before applying your color.

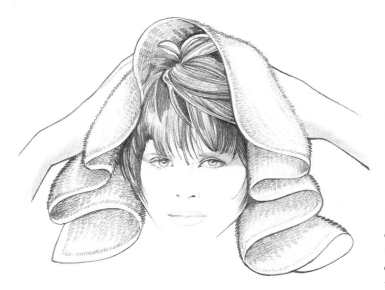

Towel dry wet hair before applying your semipermanent color to avoid diluting its optimum color impact.

Since semipermanent hair color stains the hair, it can stain the skin as well, particularly if your skin is sensitive or dry. If you do get a spot of color on your skin, a little soap and water on a facecloth will wash it right off. But don't wait too long, lest you really have to scrub your skin to remove the stain. You can exercise an ounce of prevention by applying night cream or petroleum jelly around your hair line to prevent any drips of color seeping onto your skin. Just be sure that when you wipe the cream off you don't wipe it *into* your hair!

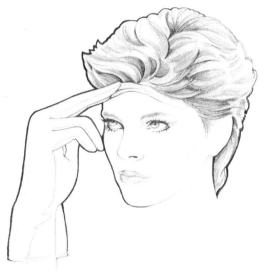

Apply a ribbon of petroleum jelly or cream to your hairline to avoid any random drips or slips.

Many semipermanent color kits contain a cap that looks like a clear plastic food storage bag with instructions to wrap it over your hair after you've applied the color. Do use it! It's meant to conserve and contain the natural heat from your body and scalp, thus encouraging better color absorption in the hair shaft. The color you apply will therefore "hold" better

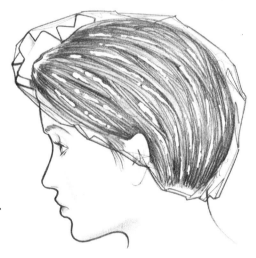

Using a clear plastic cap while color develops encourages better absorption so your color holds better.

throughout your next several shampoos. Using the cap is a matter of convenience, too. With all your hair tucked up and secured, you can go about doing other things while the color is being absorbed by your hair.

Semipermanent Color Mousses

If you're accustomed to using a styling mousse on your hair, you'll love this new way of applying semipermanent color. It's fun and very easy. Instead of the mousse adding "holding power," semipermanent mousses add color to the hair that will last through several shampoos. But since this mousse is, after all, a coloring product, resist the urge to run your fingers through your hair when you apply it as you would with a styling mousse. You want the color on your hair, not your hands. Other than that rather obvious caution, you can expect color mousses to perform just like any other semipermanent color product. Just pick your shade and mousse away.

Using Semipermanent Color to Cover Gray

If you're using semipermanent color for the first time because you're trying to cover gray, it will help to know in advance just how effective this type of hair coloring can be. It's quite simple. Successful covering of gray with semipermanent color is in direct proportion to how much gray you have.

Describing your gray hair in terms of percentages, as we did in the previous chapter, is the best way to make your evaluation. As a reminder: Five to ten percent gray means you're graying at the temples and around the front hairline; fifty percent gray or more means people you meet will refer to you as being gray-haired. The middle range, ten to thirty-five percent gray, is when you see gray appearing all the way through your hair. It's in that middle range that semipermanent color is most effective and when I recommend it most often.

Less than ten percent gray is not that noticeable and can even look distinguished. If you hate even that little gray, however, semipermanent color is a good choice for you and really will "wash the gray away." Thirty-five percent means that every third hair on your head is gray and distributed throughout the hair, making it difficult to see what your natural color really is. At the same time, while one-third of your hair has gone gray, the remaining two-thirds has most likely become drab and lost its original color impact. If that's your situation, you're at a perfect point to consider using semipermanent color, because it will do wonders to enliven your looks.

Since semipermanent color is designed to *add* color, it not only covers the existing gray in your hair, it revitalizes your natural color at the same time. Semipermanent color blends in the gray by giving both the natural color hair *and* the gray a stepped-up, colorful impression. What's more, there's a real beauty bonus involved in using this coloring method. Because any hair coloring product shows up a little lighter on gray hair, your gray is transformed into highlights of the enriched color shade you've chosen, golden glints within chestnut brown, for example, or soft ash highlights within a deeper smoky brown. You don't have to do a single extra thing to make this lovely highlighting effect happen. It occurs naturally and is one of the best reasons to use semipermanent color on partly gray hair. You can convert what may seem to be a negative (the gray) into a striking beauty bonus (sparkling highlights).

Two Ways Not *to Use Semipermanent Color*

As beautiful as semipermanent color can look when used properly, there are two mistakes that are made very frequently with this type of hair coloring. The first is picking too dark a color.

If you are using semipermanent color to cover gray, chances are the natural aging process has also left your complexion a little paler than it used to be and you've probably accumulated a few lines in your face along the way, too. Women (and men) sometimes think to themselves, "I'm going back to the hair color I had in my late teens." Recalling color accurately is something few professionals can do, much less someone without color training. And the more years in between, the less reliable your memory. Further, and most important, your face in your thirties or forties may not be up to wearing the color you had as a teenager. Going down memory lane will invariably result in your choosing a color that's too dark for you. It will create too dense a frame for your face and too harsh a contrast for your features. When choosing a semipermanent shade to cover partly gray hair, you must always go at least one shade *lighter* rather than darker if you want your hair color to look at all natural and flattering. Going a shade or two lighter means your hair will look brighter, livelier, and have more color personality.

One excellent way to tell if the semipermanent color you've chosen is too dark (besides just looking at it) is if it shampoos out too quickly—in two or three shampoos instead of the four, six, or eight the directions claim the color will last. If gray starts showing through in a week to ten days, it means you're asking too much of a hair-coloring method that's meant to refine and *add* color, not to cover more than thirty-five percent gray or to make a drastic change.

The other common mistake is to use the same shade of semipermanent color *too long.* Some women seize on one particular shade, then lock themselves into that color for *years!* What they forget is that underneath their color, they're developing more gray all the time. When some of that increased amount of gray starts to "show through," they think the color isn't holding as well as it used to and so start using their semipermanent color more often. The result is an overcoating of the hair with color that builds up, eventually making the hair look dull and lifeless, with a shoe-polish look.

At the least, you should check for the amount of gray you're developing every six months. To do this, center-part your hair in the middle of the crown (not at the temples) and, standing under good light, take a close look at your roots. If it seems every other hair is gray, you're inching up to fifty percent, which is more than the semipermanent hair-coloring method was ever designed to handle. It may be time for you to move on to permanent color, which is not a bad idea anyhow, since clinging to the same hair-color image year after year can be just plain boring. There's a great wide world of hair color out there waiting for you, and sometimes the best thing you can do for yourself is to let that old hair-color image go, and try something new and exciting.

To sum up how to avoid making semipermanent hair-color mistakes: Don't pick *too dark* a color, and don't use the same color for *too long* without checking underneath to see what's happening to your natural color.

Semipermanent Color on One Hundred Percent Gray

Let's say you've finally made it all the way to gray and you love it! Or you *almost* love it. You may find that what's bothering you is that your gray is too draining to your skin. This happens very often, and usually it's the woman whose hair has turned that beautiful blue-gray or blue-white color whose complexion begins to look very pale. In that case I suggest the smallest touch of a warmer semipermanent shade like Extra Light Beige Blonde. You only have to use it every four to six times you shampoo, but even that small amount of warming color will enliven the complexion. Your hair will still look one hundred percent gray, but with a very soft, very flattering extra dimension.

If, on the other hand, you're not thrilled with your one hundred percent gray because it is yellowish or has yellow streaks, you can easily go to one of the semipermanent products designed to eliminate the yellow and enhance your gray with silvery highlights. This is a very specialized group of products and so is not listed with the regular color shades given in the tables in chapter 8. But to give you an example, Clairol calls their product line of this type "Silk & Silver." Within the line are seven shades, ranging from Silvery Extra White for the lightest gray to Silvery Smoke for darker gray. You use this product just like any other semipermanent color—once every four to six shampoos. It may be all you need to "cool down" some of the yellow in your gray and give your hair extra shine and sparkle at the same time.

Now that you know all you need to know about using semipermanent color, whether it shampoos in (or, more accurately, shampoos *out*) or is applied with a foam or a mousse, let's sum up the high points:

SEMIPERMANENT HAIR-COLOR ADVANTAGES:
- Is a great method for beginners because it's so easy to use and so hard to make a mistake.
- Requires no retouching of the roots
- Adds color to your natural shade so your hair looks brighter and has more color impact.
- Gives you a fashion image.
- Covers gray well in the lower percentages (ten to thirty-five percent gray).
- Revives dull or faded hair and gives it more gloss and shine.
- Can "warm up" one hundred percent gray or "cool down" yellow streaks in all-gray hair.

SEMIPERMANENT HAIR-COLOR LIMITATIONS:
- Will *not lighten* the hair.
- Is not effective covering more than thirty-five percent gray.
- Should not be used more often than directions indicate or else color will build up unattractively. If color wears off too quickly, consider an alternative coloring method.

11

Highlighting Your Natural Color

Could you say any of the following?

> *"Knock on wood, I have very little gray, but I'd like to lighten my hair a little—maybe just around my face."*

> *"My own natural color is wish-washy light brown. Some highlights may be all I need."*

> *"My hair seems to be getting darker and less lively looking. I'd love to lighten things up."*

There is no such thing in nature as solid color hair. If you were to look closely at a child's blonde hair, you'd see some strands of white blonde, some gold, and some light brown. Nature always produces color within color. That is the same principle used in highlighting your own hair. Highlights are meant to imitate nature by lightening various strands of your own natural color. The effect is like a play of light shimmering through your hair. It's the difference between the way you would look standing outside on a sunny day compared with how you look on a cloudy day. Highlighting brings out the brightest color in your hair and makes it look more exciting, prettier, and more vibrant.

Highlighting Your Natural Color

The word *highlight* means many things to many people. You may describe a visit to the Uffizi Gallery as a highlight of your trip to Florence. A flaming dessert may be the highlight of a dinner party. But when it comes to hair coloring, highlights mean something very definite: They are strands that are lighter than the rest of your hair. To be even more precise, professional hair colorists define highlights this way: *Highlights are lighter strands of your overall natural hair color.*

To compare your hair to fabric, highlights create the difference between ordinary, solid-color cotton and shimmering silk gleaming in the light. The reason for this is that your eye is naturally attracted to lighter areas of a darker whole. In decorating, for example, interior designers use light to draw attention to certain details in a room. They'll use a lamp to shed extra light on a particularly beautiful table. In the theater, a lead singer will be spotlighted for a solo, even while the rest of the stage is lit. That spotlight draws the eye to the soloist. The idea behind highlighting your hair works on the same principle. Extra light draws attention to the highlighted areas, whether those areas are around your face and emphasizing certain facial features or whether the lighter highlights are scattered throughout all your hair, producing lighter areas within the darker whole.

When you highlight your hair, you do *not* change the basic color of the hair itself. You simply add extra light to your existing natural color. Thus highlighting is a coloring method that *presumes* you have plenty of natural color in your hair to begin with. If you are going gray, highlighting is *not* the best method of hair coloring for you. As a matter of fact, I don't recommend highlighting if you are more than twenty percent gray, because the gray will just mix in with the highlights and confuse the heightened color effect we're trying to produce. So let's assume your hair has lots of natural color in it and that we are pointing up that color to give the hair more glow and sparkle.

Clarifying Definitions of Highlighting, Frosting, and Streaking

For purposes of comparison and to differentiate our terms, I use *highlighting* to describe the single-step method of lightening selected strands of your own natural color hair. With this method you add more light to your hair by lightening just a *few* strands, whether around your face or here and there throughout your hair. *Frosting* is the term I use to describe the process of making your hair look blonde by lightening *many* strands all over your head, then giving those strands a color wash, which we describe in chapter 14, Frosting. Frosting requires lightening many more strands than highlighting and frosting works best as a two-step coloring method. Finally, I reserve the term *streaks* for the shocks of color you add to your hair for a disco party (see chapter 9, Temporary [Shampoo-Out] Color). Now that we're speaking the same language, let's get back to the discussion of highlighting—what happens during the lightening process and the different methods you can use to highlight your own hair.

Warm or Cool Highlights: How to Pick the Perfect Product

You really can have warm or cool highlights, depending on your color personality and which you prefer for your own hair color image. But in order to make that decision, it will help to know how hair responds to the lightening process.

All hair goes through the same stages as it is lightened. Whether you are a warm- or cool-color person makes no difference. Say your natural color is any shade of brown. When you apply a simple lightening product (one with no tint additives) to brown hair, in the first stage of lightening your hair will turn reddish brown, then it turns red, then orange, then gold, then yellow, and finally a very pale yellow. The degree of lightening depends on how dark your hair was to begin with, how strong the product is that you're using and how long you leave the product on your hair. But all hair simply being lightened goes through the same stages.

Here's the significant point: All the colors produced in the simple lightening process have a warm color hue (red, gold, or yellow). If you are a warm-color person, fine. Any of those lightened shades will suit your complexion. If that is what you're looking for, *your* product choice is a simple highlighting kit that has everything you need contained in it. Highlighting kits feature simple lightening products with no color tint additives. You mix a lightening powder with a peroxide-activated developer, apply to selected strands according to directions and there you have it.

If, however, you are a cool-color person, I want you to use a coloring product that will produce cool-color highlights. The type of product that will do this is a permanent hair-coloring preparation. You will be picking from the permanent color group that includes names like "Nice 'n Easy," "Ultress," and "Preference." Although these products are usually applied to a whole head of hair, you will be using the product on selected strands only. This type of product contains two elements you mix together: a liquid tint and a peroxide-activated developer. The beauty of using permanent color for highlighting is that it opens a broad spectrum of color possibilities and permits you to chose the *exact* color you want your highlights to be because each permanent color shade has a specific color tint in its formulation.

As for choosing the exact shade you want for your highlights, review the charts in chapter 8, Picking Your Perfect Hair Color, identify the shade name closest to your own natural color, then *choose a shade one to two levels lighter* than your own natural color. You'll see those levels listed in the "Light-to-Dark Hair-Color Shades" table, p. 110.

For example, if your hair is medium ash brown, you're at level 7. For your highlights (staying in the cool shade names), you can chose Light Ash Brown from level 6 for a very subtle effect or you can choose Dark Ash Blonde at level 5 to make your highlights a little more dramatic. If your hair is naturally Dark Ash Blonde, level 5, you can brighten and lighten your color with highlights of Medium Ash Blonde at level 4 or with Moonbeam Blonde on level 3 and so on.

The idea of using permanent hair-coloring products for your highlights may seem radical at first, but the more you think about it, the better sense it will make to you. By using permanent coloring for highlights, you dip into the broad spectrum of shades that give you wonderful control over the statement you want your hair color to make about you. If you are a cool-color person, I strongly recommend you use permanent color for your cool highlights. Even if you are a warm-color person, you'll find you can *refine* the color of your highlights by choosing an exact shade rather than just simply lightening your natural color. The choice is up to you. Now that we've discussed what shade your highlights can be, let's talk about the different methods you can use to highlight your hair.

Hair Painting with a Brush

One of the easiest ways to highlight your hair is to paint the highlights in with a brush. There are several kits on the market that contain everything

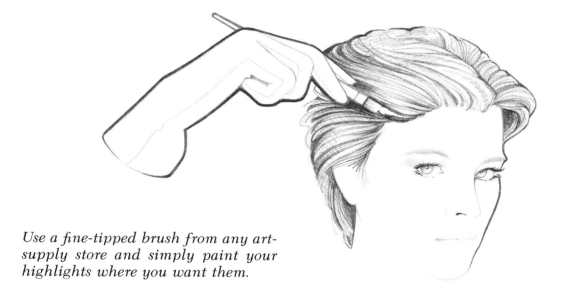

Use a fine-tipped brush from any art-supply store and simply paint your highlights where you want them.

you need to highlight your hair this way. Don't forget, though, highlighting kits offer simple lightening only. If you want your highlights in a specific shade, you'll be selecting a permanent color product and in that case, you'll need to buy your own brush. I suggest a flat-tip brush no more than one-half inch wide for painting highlights. Any art supply store will carry that type of brush and, in some cases, so will a paint store.

If your hair is wavy or worn in a layered cut, a good way to place your highlights is to stand under strong overhead light and look in the mirror to see where the light outlines your hair. That's where to paint your high-lights. If your hair is stick straight, the general area to highlight is around your face and forehead. The trick with straight hair is to create a multitude of fine highlights, particularly if your hair is on the thin side. Thin slivers of light look beautiful on this type of hair. Clumps of color do not, so keep the strands you separate to highlight skinny, skinny, skinny. And do lots of them!

Highlighting with a Comb

Another method of highlighting is to comb just enough color through your hair to create a shimmer of brighter, lighter color. This is another do-it-

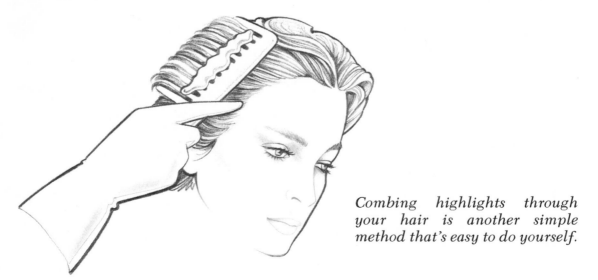

Combing highlights through your hair is another simple method that's easy to do yourself.

yourself method that's simple as can be. Start by picking the color that suits you, which, once again, will come from the permanent color product section on the shelf at your supermarket, variety, or drugstore. Mix the two elements contained in the package together, apply some of the mixture to a wide-tooth comb, then simply comb the color through your hair. Plastic or hard rubber combs are best—do *not* use a metal comb (metal can interact with hair-coloring ingredients to alter the chemical process and final color shade). The beauty of this method is particularly apparent if you usually wear your hair combed back and away from your face because that's the same way you comb the highlighting color into your hair.

Finger-Painting Highlights

This is still another method of highlighting that lets you pick the exact color you want your highlights to be. As with the comb-in method, you start by

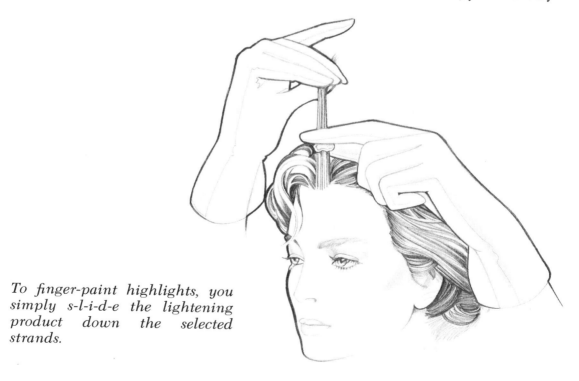

To finger-paint highlights, you simply s-l-i-d-e the lightening product down the selected strands.

selecting your permanent color product, then mix the two elements in the package together according to directions. (One extra tip: This method works particularly well with any of the new gel-type permanent colors.) Now slip on a pair of protective gloves and get ready to have the kind of fun you had as a child when you finger-painted.

Take the thinnest possible strand you can separate from the rest of your hair between your thumb and forefinger. Dip your other thumb and forefinger into the color mixture and apply a dollop of the mix to the *roots* of the strand to be highlighted. Now simply s-l-i-d-e the color down the strand. That's it! Repeat with as many strands as you like, taking care to keep the color on for the full time specified in the directions. The effect will be a frame of light shining around your face.

Where to Concentrate Highlights

Highlights give hair a glorious sparkle and glow, but there's still another benefit highlighting offers you: You can concentrate your highlights to flatter your particular face and features. The same rule that governs makeup holds for highlights: to bring forward or widen, go lighter; to recede or make narrow, go darker. The eye is naturally attracted to lighter areas, so to *direct* the eye where you want it to look, here's how to place your highlights to make the most of your face and features.

> *LONG FACE:*
> To break up the long vertical line, concentrate the highlights at the temples to widen that area and make the face look more like a classic oval. Style your hair no longer than your chin.

> *SMALL FACE:*
> Direct the eye *up* by concentrating highlights across the front crown and bangs. This will give the face more height. An extra word here: Frequently a small face goes on a short person and if you're under five feet two inches, be sure your hairstyle is no

longer than mid-neck lest it pull the eye down and make you look even shorter.

ROUND FACE:

With a face as long as it is wide, the place *not* to highlight is the temple area, which will make your face look even rounder. Leave that area dark and instead lighten just the area north of your eyebrows to give the round face a little more length. Also, you'll find an asymmetrical or side-parted hairstyle helps minimize too much roundness in the face.

SQUARE FACE:

Since the forehead, cheeks, and chin are all the same width on a square face, concentrating the highlights either at the temples or around the forehead will take the edges off a square face and aim the eye up away from the jaw. And here's a styling note: Curved bangs soften the forehead of a square face. As for an overall style, a blunt cut in which the hair swings forward of the ear, forming a curve instead of an angle, looks good against a square chin line.

HEART-SHAPED FACE:

This shape of face is also called triangular, with the bottom point at the chin. The logical area of the hair to leave *dark* is at the top, lest the forehead look even wider than it is. Extending that logic would seem to indicate that highlights belong on both sides of the jaw to widen that area, but in my opinion, this will just make those highlights look as if they've grown out too far. Thus, this face shape is the only one on which I would *not* depend on highlights for balance. Instead, look to your hairstyle and make sure it has lots of fullness and volume from the bottom of the ears on down.

PEAR-SHAPED FACE:

Narrow at the forehead, full at the cheeks and chin, this face can benefit enormously from concentrating highlights from the cheekbones up. The whole face will come into balance with liberal amounts of highlights scattered through all the hair from the top of the ears up and across the forehead. That's the same area in which to place the fullest part of your hairstyle, too. Loosely waved layers or curls across the top of the head work beautifully to bring this face shape into a pretty balance.

Too Little or Too Much?

Highlighting is one of the most subtle forms of coloring your hair because you lighten relatively few strands. But since you want to see *some* change, if you don't see enough the first time you try highlighting, *do it again!* I assume you're leaving the lightener or permanent hair-coloring product on your hair for the full time specified in the directions. But in case this is the reason you're seeing too little highlighting, set your timer and don't rinse off a minute sooner than the instructions recommend.

You might also feel you are getting too little highlighting if you were expecting too much change. Remember, this method is meant to point up your natural color by giving nature a little help in lightening certain strands so hair looks sunnier. In that sense, it's a great way to start coloring your hair because highlighting is such a subtle method. It's a turn-on for your natural hair color, but if you want or need more than that, don't expect highlighting to result in a major color change.

There's one other possibility if you are seeing too little change with highlighting, and that is you are more than twenty percent gray. As we discussed earlier, going gray involves more than developing a few gray hairs. *All* the hair becomes drabber in color. So if you're highlighting hair that is already on its way to gray, you won't get much effect from highlighting because there's not that much natural color left to serve as a base for those highlights! Over twenty percent gray, you're better off going to semipermanent or permanent hair color for your most flattering change.

At the other extreme of too little highlighting, is too much, and it can look perfectly dreadful. Too much is when the hair looks *striped* with highlights that are too light against hair that is too dark. The overall effect is one of tiger stripes, which may look great in the jungle, but can make a woman look cheap and vulgar. Highlighting is designed to be discreet, subtle, elegant, and give your hair a cared-for look. A basic rule for high-lighting is this: *Highlighting works best on hair* no darker than *medium brown.*

Redheads or dark blondes look fine with highlights, too, but if your hair is *dark* brown, highlights will look too artificial on you and you'd be better off choosing another hair-coloring technique.

Retouching Highlights

Every three or four months is about as often as you should retouch your highlights. Any more often may be too much of a good thing. When re-touching, you can simply repeat the general pattern of the highlights you used originally, but don't try to go over the exact same strands. You'll make yourself crazy, because it's virtually impossible to do, even for a profes-sional! If you completely change your hairstyle and the areas that were highlighted have disappeared, you may want to repattern your highlights. The same applies if you've cut your hair much shorter and simply cut the highlights off. In that case, use your common sense and re-highlight to dramatize the shape of your new cut.

Although highlighting is a permanent color change (it certainly doesn't shampoo out), your regrowth won't be that noticeable because you're scat-tering the lighter strands through your hair. As I've said, three to four times a year is as often as you'll have to repeat your highlighting to keep your hair looking bright and alive with a healthy glow.

To sum up everything you now know:

HIGHLIGHTING ADVANTAGES:
· Gives the hair sparkle, shine, and the look of sun streaming through it.
· Maximizes your natural color and so is perfect for young women, even teenagers.
· Can help flatter your face by concentrating light in specific areas.

- Is the perfect choice for women with less than twenty percent gray and hair that is medium brown or lighter.
- Requires retouching only three or four times a year.

HIGHLIGHTING LIMITATIONS:

- Is *not* a method for major hair-color change.
- Is not effective on hair that is more than twenty percent gray.
- Is unattractive on hair any darker than medium brown.

12
Permanent Hair Coloring

Does one of these statements apply to you?

"The first few strands of gray were interesting, but there are a lot more of them showing now and my hair is, well, no color."

"I have a successful career and a clear fashion image. I've noticed a few gray hairs, however, and have no intention of keeping them. I want to head them off at the pass."

"The dark-brown semipermanent color I've used for years suddenly looks too dark. I think I'd look better with a lighter shade."

"I've experimented with both temporary and semipermanent color and now have a good idea of what color I like best. I'm ready to take the plunge."

"My salt-and-pepper hair is nondescript and very dull. It just doesn't go with the rest of my life."

Permanent hair color offers a glorious variety of possibilities. There's a rainbow of colors waiting for you and any number of them can make you feel and look wonderfully glamorous. You can go lighter (mouse brown to ash blonde), go darker (dishwater blonde to golden-blonde), switch to another color (plain brown to rich auburn), or cover gray completely. Permanent hair color provides a galaxy of exciting choices, to help you achieve your highest beauty potential.

"New and Improved" Permanent-Color Options

Over the past two decades, manufacturers have refined their permanent coloring products to make them totally safe and easy to use. Although permanent color depends on the use of certain chemicals, these are in the mildest form they can be while still imparting color. Also, as mentioned earlier, modern hair-coloring products have formulations that are timed very accurately to be virtually mistake-proof. And further, there are so many conditioners now contained in permanent hair-coloring products that using them can make your hair look even *healthier* than it did before. And there's no doubt that permanent color gives hair the extra oomph of added body.

Perhaps the best news of all is the dramatically expanded number of shades you can choose from. Within any particular color, say medium brown, there are at least a half dozen versions available. This is not meant to confuse you, but to offer you the widest possible choice, so you can have the shade that is absolutely perfect for you. Of the marvelous variety of shades in any one color, you'll find some are more fashionable, some more conservative. Personally, I usually opt for the shade with more fashion impact, simply because I feel if you're going to color your hair, you may as well give your style image a boost at the same time. But the ultimate choice is yours, and whatever you feel you'll be most comfortable and beautiful wearing is the best shade for you.

How Permanent Color Works

Each method of hair coloring works in a slightly different way with a slightly different effect. Temporary color coats the hair with color until that color washes off. Semipermanent color stains the hair and wears off gradually. Permanent color penetrates and carries color to the very core of the hair shaft. You permanently affect the structure of the hair when using this coloring method and consequently the color you have used on your hair stays put.

This permanent color change is the result of mixing together two elements that produce a mild chemical reaction. One element is the color you've chosen, the other is the activator, or *developer,* which does just what its name suggests. When mixed with the color you've selected, it develops that color on the hair, usually by means of some type of peroxide. The hair holds this new color deep within its structure, which is why hair colored with this method *stays* that way and does not wash out. Assuming you've done some experimenting and have a good idea what color you want, permanent color is a marvelous way of establishing a signature hair color, of creating a definite fashion image, and of making a personal statement about yourself and your life-style.

While temporary and semipermanent colors are capable of increasing the color impression your hair gives, permanent color is the right choice for maximum drama and change. It helps to remember, however, that while you do *not* need retouching for either of the other two coloring methods, once you start using permanent color, you *will* have to retouch your roots to keep your hair looking picture perfect. This is the trade-off that is implicit in using permanent color: It offers you the greatest number of options and the greatest variety of shade choices, but it will require some upkeep every four to six weeks. I mention that here because I want you to make the most fully informed decision you can, taking all factors into account.

First-Time Application

If you are using permanent color for the first time on hair that has never been colored before, the application method is very simple: You shampoo it in according to directions. If your hair is tinted and you want to go darker, apply according to the directions. If you want to lighten already tinted hair, however, you must remove the old tint first. Read the instructions on whatever product you plan to use in this case, paying particular attention to any special coloring tips.

Retouching Permanently Colored Hair

Just as the shampoo-in method is the one used for your first application of permanent color, it is also one of the ways you can *retouch* your color. However, I do *not* recommend shampoo-in as the ongoing method of retouching every four to six weeks when your roots begin to show or your color needs reestablishing. Here's why. Over the months (or years), retouching by covering *all* your hair with the coloring product for the full amount of time it takes for permanent color to develop (usually 25 minutes, at least) can create too much stress on the hair and be too drying. At the most, I wouldn't want you to use the shampoo-in method of retouching permanent color more often than every second or third time you're due. The method of retouching I far prefer is the "root retouching" method in which you concentrate the permanent color on the root (regrowth) area first, then carry the color through the rest of the hair for just a few minutes. That is usually all you need to refresh and revitalize you permanent hair color. Even further, if you go to a salon to have your color retouched, you'll find that the method used almost all the time by professionals is the root retouch method. And since I want you to know how to handle your own hair like a pro, I'm now going to give you exact instructions on how to retouch your hair using the preferred root retouch method.

As long as you don't have a lot of hair spray or styling gel on the surface of your hair, it doesn't have to be freshly shampooed; a day or two later is fine. In fact, I find dry hair easier to handle when retouching. The remainder of the tips I'm about to give you describe the way I retouch hair in my salon and represent my years of experience in developing the techniques I believe work best.

1. Start by center-parting your hair from front hairline to back nape. Then part sideward over the top of your crown from the middle tip of one ear to the middle tip of your other ear. Secure each quadrant with a clip.

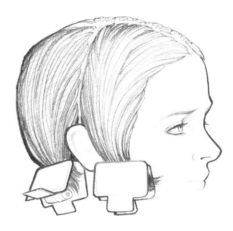

Part your hair in quadrants and secure each section with a clip.

2. Apply light face cream or petroleum jelly around the edges of your face to protect your skin from drips or slips (dry or sensitive skin absorbs color very easily).
3. Mix your two color elements according to the manufacturer's directions.
4. Slip on protective gloves.
5. Using the tip end of the applicator bottle, make your first one-eighth-inch section (back of section to front) at the top of the crown in the right front quadrant. It is extremely important that you keep each of these partings no deeper than one-eighth inch because, while hair coloring can be magical, the hair must be uniformly covered with color to achieve the desired results.
6. Holding that parted section of hair straight out from your head with your other hand, squeeze the color through the nozzle tip onto

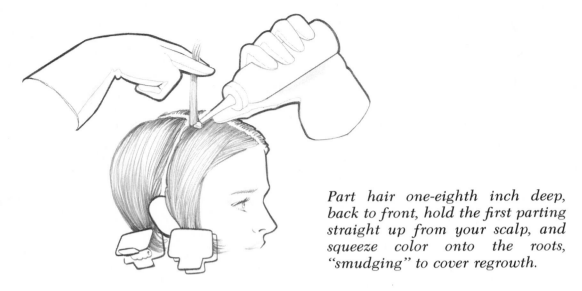

Part hair one-eighth inch deep, back to front, hold the first parting straight up from your scalp, and squeeze color onto the roots, "smudging" to cover regrowth.

the regrowth (root) area, making sure to cover the roots thoroughly.

7. Continue one-eighth-inch partings and squeezing color onto the roots this way until you have covered all the regrowth on hair in the right front quadrant. Then repeat the procedure with the left front quadrant. You'll be working on a diagonal because of the round shape of your head. Continue parting and squeezing on the right back quadrant, then the left back, until every strand of regrowth has been covered with color. Do not discard applicator bottle yet!

8. Leave all the hair loosely arranged as is. Do *not* try to "organize" your hair in a clump on top of your head or cover it with a cap. Packing the hair down in any way will intensify your body heat and cause color to develop too quickly. Instead, leave the hair open to aerate as the color develops. Now set your timer. Leave the color on the hair for the full time specified in the directions. Rinsing it off too soon is like underdeveloping film: You'll get some idea of what it's supposed to look like, but not the full impact or staying power. On the other hand, leaving the color on longer than recom-

mended serves no purpose. As we discussed, the color is designed to "shut off" automatically, so be ready for the next step as soon as your timer rings.

9. Once your roots have "taken" the color, it's time to run that color through the rest of the hair. To do this, you add between one half ounce and one ounce of *water* to the product left in the applicator bottle. If there's no product left in the bottle, add the water anyhow. Shake applicator, then apply all over the head, lightly spreading the color through all the hair. Don't rub or scrub the scalp. A light "fingertipping" is all you need. What you are doing is refreshing and restablishing your overall hair color. Wait five minutes, then take one strand, towel the color off, and check to see if the hair has reached the desired shade. If not, leave on for a few minutes more and check again. The longest you'll be leaving color on all the hair for this step is about ten minutes. Then it's on to the next step.

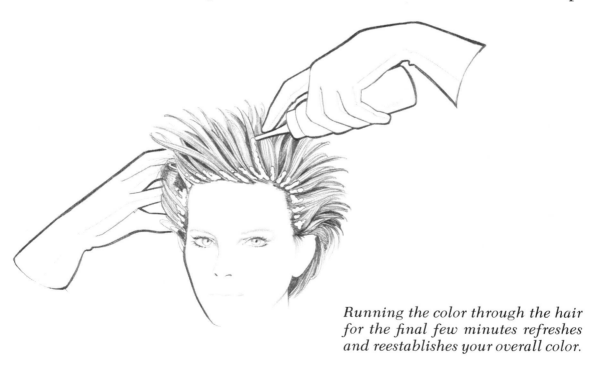

Running the color through the hair for the final few minutes refreshes and reestablishes your overall color.

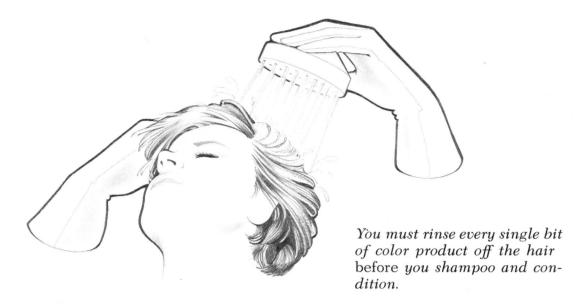

You must rinse every single bit of color product off the hair before *you shampoo and condition.*

10. Now you *rinse.* Please note, you do *not* shampoo yet, you *rinse* the color out first. It is vital that you get all of the coloring product out of the hair, so you must rinse until the water runs perfectly clear. If you shampoo prior to rinsing, you run the risk of lifting some of the color off the hair, because the cuticle is still open. Premature shampooing can result in irregular color patterns, so rinse and *then,* and only then, shampoo. Follow up with a light conditioner, and there you have it—beautifully refreshed, vibrant color!

Liquids, Cremes, and Gels

Since permanent color comes in more than one form, I want to add just a few pointers on the variety of those choices. If you have very thick hair, for example, the more liquid the form of color, the better, because it goes further. I won't make comparisons to "hamburger helpers," but liquid color does "stretch" better. Also for thick hair, when using creme hair coloring, you may find that one container may not be enough. Do be prepared with an extra package in advance. You don't want to get three quarters of the way through your one-eighth-inch partings only to find you've run out of color.

As for the newer gel forms, they are terrific to work with because they really stay put and don't run at all. Be extra careful, though, about your rinsing. Because gels stay put so well, you must be absolutely sure you've gotten all of the gel product off your hair prior to shampooing. Otherwise, excess color left on the hair will dry it out.

"Single" versus "Double" Processing

All the instructions and tips I've given you so far in this chapter have to do with what is called *single-process color*: you apply one product to the hair in one process. The single-process type of hair coloring is what I do most in my salon, but that wasn't always the case. In the 1950s and '60s there was a big demand for very light blonde shades, and many of the women who wanted that look had medium- to dark-brown hair. In order to get their hair that light, it was necessary to prebleach their hair first, then apply an appropriate tint over the lightened color. It is a two-step procedure; thus the term *double-process blonding*.

In more recent years, however, I find I'm doing less and less double-process work. These days, most women prefer a color closer to their own natural color, just brighter and prettier. For that reason, double processing isn't as fashionable as it once was. I am mentioning this method here, though, because it can be done at home, but I do not recommend it. Double processing is a very complicated method for a person without professional training to handle. If you insist on that dramatic a change in your hair color, seek out a talented professional at a salon. I've got a hunch, though, that if you were to take another look at the incredible number of hair-coloring shades available today, you would find a single-process color you'd love just as much as the double-process shade you think you want, and you'd be running less risk of doing damage to your hair.

Highlighting Permanently Colored Hair

Let's assume you've found the permanent hair-color shade that's perfect for you, have used it on your hair, and are delighted with the results. If you like, you can go even further and add some highlights. That's right. You *can* highlight permanently colored hair yourself. Highlighting on hair that is colored with this method is not difficult to do and has the effect of adding new dimension to your color. It contributes a variation and tone to your shade that is very, very pretty and gives the look of natural light shimmering through the hair. You can concentrate your highlights in front to light up your face or scatter them throughout your hair for an even more vibrant look. Highlighting permanently colored hair not only gives your shade extra believability, but when the roots grow back in, it will be less noticeable because the hair is not a solid color. Also, if you've been using the same shade for a period of time, you may be looking for a little more excitement in your color. Rather than considering the double-process method described above, consider adding some gleaming highlights to the color you already have!

There are two very different methods used to highlight hair that is permanently colored. The method you choose depends on how light or dark your shade happens to be. Let's start with the lighter range. If your hair is *medium brown or lighter,* including all the blondes, I suggest you give chapter 11, Highlighting Your Natural Color, a quick reread. The methods used to highlight permanently colored hair that is medium brown or lighter are exactly the same ones used to highlight naturally colored hair. You can finger-paint your highlights, brush them on with a fine art paintbrush, or use a comb, whichever method is most appealing to you. Don't forget, though, you'll be buying *two* products: your regular permanent color, plus a highlighting product. In choosing your highlighting shade, pick a warm- or cool-color product in keeping with your regular color product.

And here's what to look for in your highlighting product in terms of *contrast.* If your permanently colored hair is in the medium-brown range, including medium auburn, chose a *dark blonde* product for highlighting your permanent color. If your permanently colored hair is in the light-brown range, including light auburn and any of the blondes, chose a *light blonde* product to highlight your hair. What you want to do is add a play of light to your existing color—not stripes. And you can place your highlights anywhere you like, depending on your own face shape and the amount of additional "sunshine" you want to see in your hair.

Now let's talk about highlighting permanently colored hair that is *medium brown or darker,* including medium to dark auburn. Surprise! You don't use a separate highlighting product at all! You use lightweight aluminum foil. Start by separating tiny strands from the rest of your hair. You can use the straight handle of a styling comb to separate the hairs to be highlighted. Each strand should contain no more than ten to fifteen individual hairs. Now take the ten to fifteen hairs of the first strand and wrap them in a small piece of aluminum foil (approximately four inches by six inches). Start your packet one-half inch away from the scalp and be sure all the hairs are tucked securely inside the foil. Now continue separating and wrapping strands in foil until you have at least fifteen foil packets—five across the top, five on each side. You can add more if you like, too. Once you've organized all your foil packets, you proceed with your root application retouch as usual, *including* the roots of those strands enclosed in foil. At the end of your retouch procedure, run the color through the hair in the usual way for a few minutes to refresh your overall color. Keep the separate strands tucked into their packets all during this time. Rinse all the permanent color off your hair until the water runs clear. Then, and only then, do you remove the foil and shampoo as usual. That's all there is to it. Since the few strands you separated and "saved out" from the rest of the hair have had no *additional* color applied to them, they appear slightly lighter than the rest of your hair. That lightness provides a very natural-looking highlighting effect within the overall shade of the permanent color you regularly use. Isn't that easy? And the effect is really quite beautiful since it makes the hair color look so completely natural and sunny.

Just to make sure you understand highlighting permanently colored hair: Note that you incorporate any highlights in your color *after* you've established the permanent color you like best on your hair. And please, please don't double up on the two methods I've described here. Do *not* apply permanent color to certain strands, then wrap them in foil. You'll end up with chunks of broken hair plus a supremely unattractive striped effect to your color. Follow the instructions I've just given you to the letter and you'll find your hair color will look luminous, with beautiful dimension and natural depth.

Perming, "Relaxing," and Permanent Color

If you plan to perm or "relax" your hair as well as color it, do the perming or relaxing *first*. The reason for this is that all three procedures—curling, straightening, and permanent coloring—permanently affect the cuticle of the hair to which they are applied. In curling or straightening, the cuticle is lifted a little to allow more light to penetrate the hair, making the color appear lighter. Thus, if you let your permed or relaxed hair settle down for a week or so (at least two shampoos' worth), you'll get better results with your color and be better able to judge how the color will look when finished. One more tip: The ends of your hair are where normal wear and tear shows up first. If you regularly use a blow dryer or haven't had the ends trimmed recently, leave your hair color on the ends for a little less time. Otherwise, they may grab too much color.

> *PERMANENT HAIR-COLOR ADVANTAGES:*
> · Can lighten hair several shades.
> · Covers gray completely, no matter how gray you are.
> · Gives you the greatest selection of shades to choose from.
> · Adds extra "body" to the hair, a boon for fine, thin hair.
> · Provides the best choice for a fashion image.
> · Since it doesn't shampoo out, it offers a "signature" shade you can call your own.
>
> *PERMANENT HAIR-COLOR LIMITATIONS:*
> · Requires root retouching every four to six weeks.

13

Leslie Blanchard's Favorite Salon Formulas

As you've seen in the previous chapter, permanent hair coloring is the method that gives you the greatest number of color options, no matter how drab or gray your hair may be to begin with. Permanent coloring is the method I use most often in my New York salon because it lets me play with the color more and customize each woman's individual shade to suit her perfectly. Sometimes I'll vary the impression a particular color gives by adding highlights, a technique I also described in chapter 12, Permanent Hair Coloring. But to tell you the *whole* truth, sometimes I go *beyond* highlighting when I want to create a special shade. Sometimes I mix *two* permanent colors together to accent a particular aspect of a shade. I may want to make it a little lighter, a little brighter, redder, or blonder. If you've been using one color for some time, feel confident handling hair color, and want to vary your color just a bit (a smidge lighter in summer, warmer in winter), the advanced technique I'm about to describe may be one you'd like to try.

I told you at the beginning of this book that I would share all my tricks of the trade with you and that's just what I'm about to do. I'm now giving you my own tried-and-true salon formulas, the ones I've developed over the years. I use them all the time because they are wonderful classics and never disappoint me.

Let's clarify just a few points, however, right here at the beginning. These formulas are for hair that is permanently colored *only*. There's no point in getting this inventive with your coloring if the resulting shade simply washes out as it does with temporary color or gradually wears off as it does using the semipermanent method of coloring.

Point 1: These formulas are designed for use with permanent hair color *only*.

Point 2: You'll be mixing *two shades* together. That means you will be *buying two packages* off the shelf. In choosing your two colors, you *must* stay with the same manufacturer and the same brand name of color. *No crossing over brands or product lines!* For example, if you're using L'Oreal's "Preference," both packages you buy should have the same brand name. Don't mix "Preference" with "Excellence." Same with Clairol. Your two shades should *both* be "Nice 'n Easy" or whatever other Clairol-brand product you select. You're being creative enough by mixing your own color. Don't push your luck by attempting to be a professional chemist as well!

Point 3: Measure carefully. In all the formulas that follow, I've divided each into *thirds*: two parts basic color, one part accent color. Most permanent color products come in two-ounce containers (two ounces of color, two ounces of developer). But for these formulas, you will be mixing *three* ounces of color (two ounces of basic color plus one ounce of accent color) with *three* ounces of developer (you always mix in equal parts, color to developer). This means that in addition to buying two packages of color, you'll have to buy an applicator bottle that holds *six* ounces of mixture. These bigger size applicators are not hard to find, though. Large drug stores carry them, as do beauty supply shops.

The two packages of permanent color you'll be buying will give you a total of four onces of color and four ounces of developer when you'll only need three ounces of each. Can you keep the leftover ounce of accent color and the leftover ounce of developer for your next retouch? Yes, you can, so long as you haven't mixed the color with the developer (this procedure sets off an irreversible chemical reaction and that mixture *cannot* be stored), and so long as you cap each of the two containers tightly and store in a cool, dry place.

In giving you these salon formulas, I do not mean in any way to imply that you won't get great results from using a single color. You will! What I'm offering you here are some advanced variations for those of you who have been coloring your hair for a while and feel comfortable with the procedure. All the shade names of my salon hair-coloring formulas correspond to the same names used in our tables in chapter 8.

TO ACHIEVE	MIX TOGETHER
Light "cool" blonde	two parts Extra Light Ash Blonde with one part Medium Ash Blonde
Medium "cool" blonde	two parts Medium Ash Blonde with one part Light Ash Blonde
Dark "cool" blonde	two parts Medium Ash Blonde with one part Dark Ash Blonde
Light "warm" blonde	two parts Extra Light Beige Blonde with one part Sunbeam Blonde
Medium "warm" blonde	two parts Sunbeam Blonde with one part Light Beige Blonde
Dark "warm" blonde	two parts Sunbeam Blonde with one part Dark Golden Blonde
Light reddish blonde	two parts Honey Blonde with one part Reddish Blonde
Medium reddish blonde	two parts Reddish Blonde with one part Bright Copper
Light auburn	two parts Bright Copper with one part Lightest Auburn
Medium auburn	two parts Medium Auburn with one part Light Auburn
Dark auburn	two parts Medium Auburn with one part Dark Auburn

TO ACHIEVE	MIX TOGETHER
Light "cool" brown	two parts Dark Ash Blonde with one part Light Ash Brown
Medium "cool" brown	two parts Light Ash Brown with one part Medium Ash Brown
Dark "cool" brown	two parts Medium Ash Brown with one part Dark Ash Brown
Light "warm" brown	two parts Honey Blonde with one part Light Golden Brown
Medium "warm" brown	two parts Light Golden Brown with one part Medium Golden Brown
Dark "warm" brown	two parts Medium Golden Brown with one part Dark Golden Brown

In each of the formulas above, we've amplified the light play in each shade to give it a very special dimension. As you know by now, there is no such thing in nature as solid-color hair. That's why these formulas look as natural as they do. All have a special color texture and extra depth that make the hair color very *believable*.

Note that if you are covering more than fifty percent gray, all the formulas listed here will show up one level *lighter*. Gray hair has no pigment per se, so any color you use on top of it will show up very quickly and will seem brighter as well. So, if you want to be a light "warm" blonde, use the *medium* "warm" blonde formula given here, for example. If you're going for a medium "cool" brown, try the *dark* "cool" brown formula, and so forth.

This is an advanced technique for experienced home hair colorists, but as with any hair coloring, I don't want you to be unpleasantly surprised by the results. Whatever you do, *don't* skip the strand test we described in chapter 7. Snip a strand of your hair, apply the color mixture, let it dry, and hold the tinted strand against your skin to be absolutely *sure* you're happy with the shade before proceeding.

Warming Up "Cool" Color

And here is a final, final piece of professional advice that is *critical* for those of you who diagnosed yourselves cool-color persons back in chapter 8. It has to do with the loss of natural color pigment in both your hair and your skin. *If you are a cool-color person more than fifty percent gray and/or over forty years old, you must add some warm color to your cool formula.*

Here's why. If your hair is fifty percent gray or more, to take the first point, more than half your hair has lost all of its natural pigment. Since gray hair has no trace of red or gold in it (as *all* naturally pigmented hair does, whatever its shade), gray hair possesses no warmth whatsoever. Putting a completely cool color over gray makes your hair look *extra* cool and unnatural. Hair that retains at least some of its natural pigment still has some warmth and glow when you color it; the final shade has depth and dimension because of the warmth shining through from underneath—like painting over a warm-beige wall. But with pigmentless gray hair, a formula that contains no warmth at all will give the hair a cold, almost metallic quality —like that of a white wall painted "aluminum." To give you just one example: If you are more than fifty percent gray and use a hair-coloring formula that is one hundred percent Ash Blonde, your hair will take on a flat, shadowy look that is never, never flattering. To avoid that cold look, all you have to do is to add a warm-color accent to your cool formula. That warm accent does wonders in making your final shade look pretty and *believable*!

Even further, loss of natural pigment occurs with more than your hair. When you're over forty, your *skin* loses some of its natural pigment, too. As we age, our complexions normally begin to look a bit paler and less rosy. For the cool-color person, that loss of pigment becomes a crucial consideration in developing a personal hair-color formula. Putting one hundred percent cool hair color against skin that has already begun to lose its natural pigment will make your complexion look absolutely ashen! You'll look exhausted all the time. Even if you don't have that much gray in your hair, after forty you *must* give your complexion a break and add a warm shade to your hair color; it should be at least one-third of the total amount used. That touch of warmth in your hair will "spill over" onto your skin, giving your complexion a fresh, vibrant look.

As you can see, adding warmth to an all-cool hair-color formula has the effect of reinstating, reestablishing, and *restoring* natural warm pigment in both the hair *and* the complexion. If you are a cool-color person with fifty percent gray or more, *or* a cool-color person over forty, adding a warm-color accent to your formula is one of the best things you can do for your looks.

Now let's get on with the actual formulas. Listed below are a series of essentially cool hair-color shades that incorporate a touch of that all-important warmth. You'll recognize the shade names because they are the same ones I've used earlier in this chapter and the same ones that appear in the tables in chapter 8, Picking Your Perfect Hair Color. Do note that these formulas are limited to cool blondes and cool browns. Warm blondes and browns, plus the reds and auburns, are all warm shades to begin with and as such would not be the primary color direction a cool-color person would take. So for all of you cool-color women over forty or with fifty percent or more gray, here's how to mix your hair-color formula to include that vital, flattering touch of warmth.

TO ACHIEVE	MIX TOGETHER
Light cool blonde with a warm accent	two parts Extra Light Ash Blonde with one part Sunbeam Blonde
Medium cool blonde with a warm accent	two parts Medium Ash Blonde with one part Light Beige Blonde
Dark cool blonde with a warm accent	two parts Medium Ash Blonde with one part Dark Golden Blonde
Light cool brown with a warm accent	two parts Dark Ash Blonde with one part Light Golden Brown
Medium cool brown with a warm accent	two parts Light Ash Brown with one part Medium Golden Brown

Dark cool brown with a warm accent	two parts Medium Ash Brown with one part Dark Golden Brown

Please understand that adding this much of a warm accent to your cool-color formula does *not* make your hair look totally warm. All it does is to give your final shade more depth and lend more life to your skin. It also makes your hair look shiny and produces a very believable color. And no—that touch of warmth will not affect your wardrobe color choices or throw your color image off. You'll stay within your basic color palette, but your hair color will simply have a bit more dimension. As far as cosmetics are concerned, you'll still look terrific in all your pinks, lavenders, violets, and mauves. If anything, you may find that because your entire appearance is brighter and livelier, you may want to brighten your lipstick and blusher, too.

You may be amazed, in fact, to see the difference simply adding a small amount of warmth to your cool-color formula truly makes in your overall appearance. Your hair will look fresh and flattering, and the spillover effect that warmth creates on the skin provides the difference between an older woman looking cold or tired and that same woman looking fresh, energetic, and vital. Believe me. I'm giving you the real inside story here. I've seen thousands of women walk out of my salon looking as if they've just had a facial and are wearing fresh makeup when all we've done is warm up their hair color a little. Adding that touch of warmth to an all-cool color formula is one of the best secrets of professional hair coloring that I can give you. Take my "warm-up" advice to heart as you customize your own hair-color formula. Don't forget, I want you to look your radiant best at all times.

14
Frosting

Does one of these statements describe your hair-color situation?

> *"I thought I'd like a few highlights, but my hair doesn't look different enough. I want more."*

> *"I love the look of blonde hair, but absolutely refuse to deal with retouching every four to six weeks."*

> *"I've used shampoo-out color, but am ready for something much lighter."*

If you're looking for a hair-color change that produces a "wow" response, this is it! Frosting not only gives you the illusion of being blonde, it creates instant glamour and sophistication. While highlighting concentrates lighter strands around the face, frosting carries that flattering light play through all the hair. And although the term *frosting* has been around for years, there's nothing old-fashioned or dated in looking like a woman who is pampered and cared for, because frosting *looks expensive*!

While I don't usually associate hair coloring with any particular age group, somehow frosting on a very young woman in her teens or early twenties looks too precocious. She's usually better off with some pretty highlighting. But for the woman who knows who she is and who possesses an aura of sophistication, frosting looks absolutely wonderful and beautifully appropriate. It's as if the dimensional aspect of frosting with its lighter strands weaving through the hair matches the dimensional personality of the confident woman wearing it. She knows she can carry almost anything off well, and her frosted hair looks as if it matches her personality perfectly.

Frosting: All or Nothing

While frosting and highlighting share the same easy upkeep, there is one very important difference between the two. You can spot highlights just around your face, but if you want the overall blonde look frosting can produce, it's *all or nothing.* You must carry frosting all the way through your hair to create a blonde image, front, center, and back. Otherwise your hair may look as if you were interrupted in the middle of coloring it, or that you started to go blonde and then changed your mind. Also, if you want the blonde illusion frosting offers, be aware that it may take you a little more time than some other coloring methods to do properly. Still, it will be well worth that extra effort when you see the transformation frosted hair can make in your looks.

Frosting with a Kit

Most hair-coloring manufacturers have a frosting kit that includes the lightening product, a full head cap that ties under your chin, and a plastic crochet hook with which you pull strands through holes in the cap for color application. Most of the caps I've seen have been very well designed and the spacing of the holes has been well thought out. Also, the cap usually has a round shape that curves nicely against the shape of your head. The cap method of frosting is, without question, the best and most *foolproof* method to use when frosting your hair at home, because it shows you exactly which strands to pull through for lightening, so your frosting will be evenly distributed throughout your hair. As you might guess, however, I have several frosting tips of my own I'd like to pass along to you, as well as some advice on which shade of "blonde illusion" will look best on you and how to produce that exact shade when frosting your own hair.

Picking a "Regular" or "Extra-Light" Frosting Kit

Some frosting kits come with a lightener that has been formulated in a lesser or greater degree of strength. You'll see them described as "regular frosting" or "extra-light frosting" or words like that. The implication is that if you have very dark hair you will need a stronger lightening product to create the desired frosting effect. For my money, that's exactly the look to *avoid!* If you have very dark hair and use a maximum lightening product for frosting, you'll end up with hair that's striped like a tiger's fur. That look, as I've mentioned before, may look great on a jungle cat but is the antithesis of elegance and sophistication. Bold stripes are too jarring to the eye. Consequently, for the woman with dark hair I recommend a "regular" frosting kit because while the selected strands will be definitely lighter, they won't be so extreme as to look unnatural. If you have medium-brown hair or lighter, however, the "extra lightening" kit may be fine. Do be careful, though, not to set up such an extreme contrast between your frosted strands and your natural color that you develop a "shadow" at the roots; it can make your hair look as if it's ready for retouching two weeks after you've frosted it. One final point to keep in mind: "Extra-light" on a frosting kit means extra *fast.* Keep checking to be sure your hair isn't getting too light, and if you've permed or precolored your hair, remember that it will get lighter faster using the accelerated version of a frosting product. If you're still unsure of which type of kit to use, go for the more conservative "regular" frosting variety no matter what your natural hair color. At least that way you won't be going too far with your frosting.

Strand Selection: How Much, How Many

Once you have the cap on your head, there are several decisions you can make as to how much frosting you want.

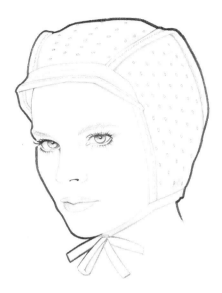

You can control the amount of frosting you like by drawing strands through every hole or every other hole.

If this is the first time you've ever tried lightening your hair, you may want to pull strands of hair through every *other* hole. If your hair is fairly thick, though, even if you're a beginner, you'll be better off using *every single hole* on the cap; the more hair you have, the more strands you'll need lightened in order to establish the blonde illusion of frosting. Where the cap can't be beat is in guiding you through an even pattern of frosting certain strands all over your head.

When picking out the strands to be frosted, here is a very good guideline: *The closer to the face, the finer the strands should be.*

When working those fine strands through the holes in the cap, wiggle the tip of the crochet hook a little to drop the extras and draw out no more than about ten to fifteen individual hairs through each hole in the cap. This is the most important part of the frosting process! Take your time, but make sure the strands nearest your face are as fine as possible.

Even more important, if you have very fine hair, you must be *extra* careful making each strand you pull out very delicate because with this type of hair, every single strand shows up very clearly. Whatever your hair

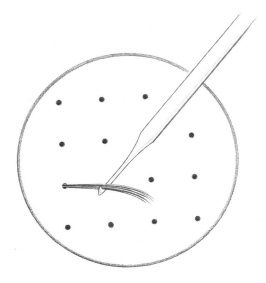

The strands near your face should be as fine as possible—no more than ten to fifteen hairs each.

type, though, the way your hair looks around your face is what gives it a pretty frame. It's also what other people see first, so you want that area to look extra-specially perfect. Once you have all your strands picked out, it's time for the next step.

Applying the Lightener

When mixing the lightening product, mix it slowly and make sure it's not too wet. What you're looking for is a paste consistency that is easy to handle and will give you more control. When applying the lightening product to the strands, start at the *back first.*

The strands around your face are more delicate and are inclined to lighten more quickly, so to make your lightening consistent all over your head, start at the back where hair is naturally darkest. Continue applying the lightener until all the strands are covered, then set your timer. When the appropriate number of minutes has elapsed, rinse the color off *while still wearing the cap.* You must get all the lightener off the hair. Then and only then do you remove the cap, shampoo, and condition.

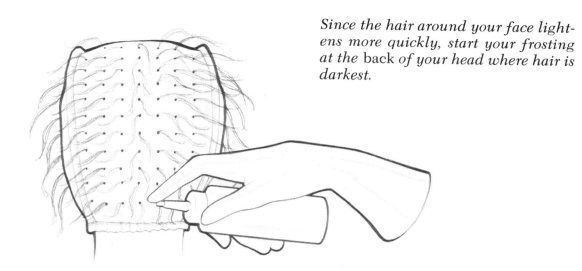

Since the hair around your face light-ens more quickly, start your frosting at the back *of your head where hair is darkest.*

If you like the way your new frosting looks, wonderful! You don't have to do another thing. For those of you who want an even more sophisticated look to your frosting, however, I'd like to explain how to give your light-ened strands a "color wash." It's a professional technique but it's not hard to do and, to my eye, has the effect of customizing your frosting so it becomes your own personal hair-color signature. Also, as far as I'm con-cerned, taking this second color step is the maximum preferred method of frosting.

The Color-Wash Follow-Up to Frosting

As you know by now, all hair lightens in the same stages, from red to orange to yellow. Since these are all golden hues, they suit the warm-color person quite well. If you are a cool-color individual, however, and are frosting your hair, you may want to give your lightened strands a cool-color finish to add a final, flattering emphasis to your frosting and to your face.

What you'll need for a color wash is a container of permanent color and some developer to mix with that color. You know all about selecting the right shade by now. For reminder: To make a cool-color wash you'll be picking a permanent color that has "ash," "moon," "silver," "smoke," or "cool" in its name. And in this case, you should choose a shade that is the lightest in its category, Extra Light Ash Blonde, for example. Here's the formula for a color wash:

> one part permanent color
> one part developer
> one part water

That's right. *Water.* You *dilute* the coloring product. Shampoo this formula into the wet hair and leave on for two or three minutes—*no more.* Then rinse out right away and rinse again, then shampoo and condition. That's all there is to it. Because the color wash is diluted and stays on the hair for a brief two to three minutes, only the strands you have lightened will pick up any of the extra color. And a color wash will not lighten the hair any further. All it does is to *refine* the color in your already lightened strands and impart a richer color tone to the strands you've frosted.

I've been describing a color wash for the cool-color person, which is when I recommend it most often. But if you are a warm-color person, you too can benefit from adding the extra dimension of a color wash to your frosting (Jan Kennedy in chapter 2 is a good example). For you, shades in the honey, sunlit, or beige range are what to look for, and again, choose the lightest gold or the lightest honey for your permanent color element. Customizing your color this way will give an extra dimension of *warmth* to your newly frosted hair.

I know this particular technique is not for everyone. It requires buying a frosting kit, permanent color, and developer, and it makes frosting a two-step method. But I promise you, if you follow up your frosting with a color wash just once, you'll see immediately why professionals do it this way. The hair's lightened streaks are integrated into a rich color effect that is very individual, very striking, very beautiful, and very elegant.

Frosting Partially Gray Hair

If your hair is on its way to gray, but has not gone beyond twenty-five percent, frosting can be a very good method for you to use to dramatize your hair color. There's only one thing you have to be extra careful about, though, and that is leaving the lightener on the selected strands until they get very light, almost as pale as your gray.

In this situation, I heartily recommend using the "extra light" frosting kit. I have another suggestion for frosting partially gray hair, too. I strongly recommend that after you lighten the selected strands according to the directions in your kit, you take a second step and give your hair a rinsing of color. This second step could be the color wash described above using permanent color, it could be a semipermanent shampoo-out shade, or it could even be a temporary rinse. What I want to see is those strands you have lightened combined with your gray to produce an overall effect in a *specific shade.* If you leave the lightened strands to go it alone, they will look pale yellow. Then there's your gray. That is not a pretty mix. What *will* be pretty is an overall color statement in "moonbeam" or "sunlit" frosting that uses those lightened strands *plus* your gray to create your own personal color statement. Once you have that color established, all you have to do is keep the hair beautifully conditioned to look smooth, shining, and lustrous at all times.

Retouching Frosted Hair

Let's say you've frosted your hair and are thrilled with the new blonde impression you've created for yourself. Stop right there. The biggest mistake made with frosting is doing too much of it. Your reasoning may be that if it looks good now, it will look even better blonder. Not true. Frosting is meant to *vary* the amount of light filtering through your hair, thus giving it a dimensional glow. When you lighten too much, the hair goes over the edge and begins to put a drain on your good looks instead of enlivening them. Also, if you lighten too many strands, you'll start looking *completely* blonde, except for your dark roots. If you want that all-blonde look, think about permanent color, not frosting.

Overfrosted hair is most apparent on women with medium to long hair and shows up most quickly on hair that is straight, fine, and/or worn in a smoothly combed style. If that describes your hair and your hairstyle, be particularly careful not to overfrost. Providing you haven't taken your frosting too far, you should have to retouch only three or four times a year. And as with highlighting, don't even try to go over the same strands you frosted before. It's impossible to isolate them. Proceed as you did the first time you frosted. Your newly refreshed, frosted hair will give you an elegant, cared-for look.

FROSTING ADVANTAGES:
· Gives a dramatic, blonde impression.
· Makes a statement of elegant, expensive-looking hair color.
· Can be followed up with a second quick color wash that customizes your hair color and creates a personal color signature.
· Lets you control how blonde you want to be.
· Is a good method to use if you're partially gray (twenty-five percent or less).
· Requires retouching only three or four times a year.

FROSTING LIMITATIONS:
· Not recommended for very young women or those with more than twenty-five percent gray.
· May require a second color step to produce a cool frosting effect.
· May need another color step if you're frosting partially gray hair.

15
When Not to Do It Yourself

Can you say any of the following?

> *"My hair is very dark, but there's a movie-star blonde inside me dying to get out."*

> *"I've been coloring my hair at home for years, but it just doesn't look right to me anymore."*

> *"I've gone too far with blonding my own hair. It's breaking off in places and sticking out all over."*

I truly believe that home hair coloring is one of the greatest beauty advances of our time. Millions and millions of dollars have been spent inventing and refining home hair-color products to make them easy to handle and predictable to use. The number of shades you can choose from has expanded to a staggering number of possibilities, so much so that there is no such thing as bad hair coloring, just bad choices as to what will suit you best. What's more, home hair-coloring products have been meticulously tested over and over again before you ever see them on the shelf. I trust these products and enthusiastically recommend them to you.

But even I have to admit that there are some situations in which you'd be better off going to a salon for professional help. Sometimes all you may need is an objective opinion or a word of encouragement. Frequently, the women I talk to aren't that far away from where they should be with their color. They just need an official endorsement that the direction they've taken is the right one for them. Then again, there are cases in which hands-on help is the only practical solution, when hair has been overcolored, overprocessed, and is breaking off in chunks. Seeking the help of a professional in those instances is like going to a doctor when you know something is seriously wrong, compared with going to the drugstore for a quick headache remedy. What a real professional can do is to start you off immediately on a series of treatments that will get your hair through that transitional stage until it has recovered sufficiently to begin in a healthier, new direction. There are several situations in which I advise you *not* to do it yourself, but to seek professional help.

Radical Change

Making a dramatic, radical change in your looks is a classic case of when you should get yourself to a good salon. Say that in your heart of hearts, you want to be a very light blonde. Although I may not personally agree with that objective in nine out of ten cases and would suggest a pretty, single-process blonde shade instead, that tenth woman might just look wonderful with shimmering, pastel-blonde hair, particularly if she has gorgeous skin. Getting her hair that light will involve double-process blonding, a method in which hair is prelightened, then toned in a particular shade. As I mentioned in chapter 12, Permanent Hair Coloring, trying to do this at home involves too wide a margin for error and too much potential for doing damage to the hair. Double-process blonding is a method that belongs in a salon where a professional can keep a careful, watchful eye on the lightening and toning of your hair. With that type of close supervision, you'll be assured that no damage is being done and that your final color will be the perfect pale blonde you've always dreamed of having.

Another situation in which double-process blonding might be recommended is if you have salt-and-pepper hair—when your hair looks as light as it is dark, with neither the dark nor the gray predominating. In order to make salt-and-pepper hair come out with some color uniformity (no matter what actual shade), it may be necessary to prelighten the dark gray to bring it into better balance with the light gray, then enrich *all* the hair with a warm or cool final shade. Sometimes permanent color used at home will do the trick and will give you all the color you want. But if you've already tried that and have not been pleased with the results, it's time for professional help.

The Professional Consultation

Sometimes all you need at a salon may be a consultation. Say you're not sure if the color you're using at home is the best possible choice for you. That is a good reason to check in with a professional colorist. You'll not only get an opinion of how your hair looks now, you'll get some ideas of how else you could be coloring it, including options you may not have even considered. You may need a little more direction and that's all. You may need a lot more, and the professional will give you that advice, too. Be aware, though, that you don't have to follow the advice given to the nth degree. What you're getting is a recommendation, not the Eleventh Commandment! If you're not comfortable with what you hear, get a second opinion!

In general, I'm a great believer in the professional hair-coloring consultation, so much so that I give them all the time. No woman in my New York salon has her hair *touched* without having had a personal consultation with me first. And I charge for those consultations. When a woman comes in for a consultation I charge twenty-five dollars for my advice on what I think she should do with her hair. At other salons throughout the country the fee can vary and is usually deductible from any subsequent services, just as it is in my salon. I mention this so you'll understand why there may be a charge for a consultation. When I give one, I don't hold anything back. I give every woman I talk to first-rate advice on how her hair can and should look. Further, I tell her exactly what choices she has and what type of maintenance each requires, so she not only knows what to do, she knows how to follow through, so she'll be comfortable living with her new color. If she then wants to take that advice and go somewhere else to have it done or try it herself at home, fine!

That's exactly what I'm doing in this book, giving you all the best advice I can so you can do it yourself, and this book costs *less* than a consultation, so you have a bargain in your hands!

The reason I feel so strongly about the consultation is that I really want you to know all you possibly can about looking your very best, whether I'm talking to you in person or through this book. Whatever you take away from a consultation, there is one central point and purpose to that conversation: to create the appropriate, flattering direction your hair color should take. With that in mind, it's helpful for you to understand this: *It is much more difficult to create beautiful hair color than it is to maintain it.* That's why I feel so strongly about your getting the best advice you can before setting your color course.

When you arrive for your consultation, feel free to bring pictures of a hair color you think might look good on you. Just be sure to narrow the selection first. If you bring all blonde pictures, for example, you show you've already focused to some degree. Then the colorist can take it from there.

As far as finding the right person to color your hair, or even to consult with, word of mouth is still the best reference by far. Knowing the profession as I do, I'd be sure to look for someone who does *at least* as much color as he or she does cuts. Ideally, the person would do nothing *but* color, but outside of New York and other large cities, those professionals are few indeed. Talk to friends and friends of friends and you'll find the right person.

Damaged Hair

Beyond going to a professional for double-process blonding or a consultation, there are a few other situations in which you're better off not doing it yourself. Dealing with already damaged hair is a prime example. I have seen many women who have tried double-process blonding on their own and made a mess of it. I've have cautioned you already against doing that. In the vast majority of cases, the woman who clings to double-process blonding hasn't taken a new look at the improved products and shades available to her in the '80s. Chances are she can get just as pretty a shade with half the wear and tear on her hair, and update her image at the same time. So don't get stuck with a color process that imperils the health of your hair.

Another source of hair damage is the curling iron or wand. Unlike electric rollers that cool off once they're in the hair, a curling wand stays hot, hot, hot. And when it's used over and over again on a daily basis, I promise you it will damage your hair. Still another damage condition occurs when you perm your hair too often. Perms are a great boon to your beauty image, but they were never designed to be used every eight weeks! To avoid overperming, don't repeat the process any more often than every three to four months, and then try to concentrate on the roots, or regrowth area, only.

In almost every case of damaged hair I see, some part of the damage is due to not having used a conditioner often enough, particularly on hair that is exposed to the elements (or a chlorinated pool) on a regular basis. I'll tell you more about taking care of your color-treated hair in the next chapter, but for now, know how to head off damage: deep-condition regularly. Conditioning will not make the hair too soft. What it will do is strengthen the hair shaft, give it more elasticity, and beautify your hair color. As a matter of fact, one of the most frequent prescriptions I give to women with damaged hair is a series of deep-conditioning treatments. They make up for all those times you didn't condition at home, to start with. But even more important, these treatments get the hair back into a condition in which it can begin to restore itself to health. During that time, I let nature take its course. I do *not* try to recolor hair that is damaged until it has grown out to the point where there is more healthy hair to deal with than damaged hair. So keep that in mind and don't let your hair get to a damaged state before seeking professional help.

One last point about hair that begins to look less than its best: Hair is an eerily accurate barometer of what else is going on in your life. Stress, physical exhaustion, emotional pressures all show up in your hair. Sometimes even before any other physical symptoms occur, your hair will begin to look just a little drab, a little "off." This can mean it's time you took a real vacation! Hair that looks as if it's lost all its energy is a very good warning that trouble is brewing in other areas of your life. Please don't ignore that signal.

Color Buildup

If you've been using semipermanent color for years (the type that gradually shampoos-out) and have stayed with the same shade all that time, there's a good chance your hair may be suffering from color buildup. When this happens, hair appears too dark and very dull, with a waxy, shoe-polish look to it. In order to get shine and flattering dimension back into your color, the buildup will have to be removed and your shade recalculated to a more appropriate color. The corrective method for lifting excess color off your hair can be done at home, but there's less of a gamble involved if you have it done professionally. Further, readjusting your color after removing previous buildup must be done very carefully. That's why I recommend you take yourself to a salon for professional problem solving if your shampoo-out color has become too dark. The up side is that you may emerge with a gorgeous new hair-color shade you hadn't considered before. There is so much wonderful hair color out there, you shouldn't settle for anything less than sensational.

Cost Efficiency

Going to a salon instead of doing your hair yourself doesn't always have to be because you've developed a problem. You could choose to have your hair done professionally because it's cost efficient for you to do so. If you run your own business or are a high-priced executive, having someone else do your hair may end up costing less than if you spent the time doing it yourself. Most executive women I know are keenly aware of how the money they earn breaks down in terms of dollars per hour. Frequently, going to a salon ends up being *less* expensive for them in the long run.

While we're on the subject of costs, let me suggest that you ask, in advance of your appointment, exactly what it will cost to have your hair done at a salon. How much is charged for a haircut, for single-process color, for highlighting? How much for blowing dry your hair? Is conditioning after the shampoo extra? If so, how much? Salons charge according to how much *time* each procedure takes, particularly with hair color. Temporary color that is simply rinsed through the hair is the least expensive. Frosting is the most expensive. Picking out all those fine strands, lightening, and then toning them requires the most time of any hair-coloring method, and so it costs the most. But since you have to have it done only three or four times a year, the cost can be amortized over a longer period.

Time Efficiency

If you are a housewife with growing children, it may be *time* efficient for you to carve salon hours out of your schedule, reserving that time for yourself and for having your hair done properly. Otherwise, you may find yourself trying to do your own color on an installment plan: half now, half later. This is a disastrous way to attempt hair color which *must* be done, start to finish, all at one time. Snatching twenty minutes here or there is no way to approach coloring your own hair. You give yourself short shrift trying to cram a beauty procedure into odd moments.

Another reason to seek professional help for time efficiency is if you are in a deadline-oriented business where every second counts. Barbara Walters, whose interviews and on-air time are tightly scheduled, is one example. Helen Gurley Brown, the editor of *Cosmopolitan* magazine, is another.

If you, like them, are constantly cramming every hour with ninety minutes' worth of activity, you're best off taking a taxi to a salon, having your hair done perfectly, and getting on to your next appointment.

Feeling Good

There's one more reason I'd suggest as a good one for having your hair done professionally. It's totally emotional: because you *want to.* It's a treat to have someone else do for *you,* rather than always having to do everything yourself. It's nice to be pampered. Having someone massage your temples and the back of your neck while shampooing your hair is wonderfully relaxing. Having someone blow-dry your hair with rhythmic precision is another nice feeling. Looking in the mirror when your hair is finished and knowing you didn't have to raise a finger to look so pretty is a wonderful feeling, too. So if you need a lift, or simply want to be taken care of a little, take yourself to a salon and put yourself in the hands of a professional. It will be as good for your mental health as it will be for your hair.

16
Taking Care of Color-Treated Hair

Would you describe your hair any of these ways?

"My hair looks great when I first color it, but then it gets very brassy."

"I tint my hair regularly and love it, but I find it very difficult to comb after shampooing."

"My hair is both permed and colored, but when I blow it dry, it gets very fuzzy and flyaway."

"Wearing a hat in the sun to protect my hair color is just too much bother."

"My hair color looks terrific in the winter, but once summer comes it fades very quickly. I play a lot of tennis, particularly singles, and wonder if perspiration is affecting my color."

"My highlighted hair gets so limp, it just sticks to my head and stays there."

Hair color is one of life's great pleasures. It brightens, beautifies, and does wonders for the way you appear to others and the way you feel about yourself. Once you start to use hair coloring, however, you must be willing to maintain it at its best if you want to continue dramatizing your own good looks. When I say "maintain" I don't mean just regular retouching, which is important, too. What I mean is day-to-day caring for your color-treated hair in the same way you care for your skin on a daily basis to keep it looking moist and pretty. Think of your hair as a beautiful flowering plant; the more you care for it every day, the longer it keeps blooming and rewarding you with its beauty.

Choosing the Right Shampoo

The first item to consider in treating tinted hair well is choosing the right shampoo. Some are simply too strong and actually strip color off the hair, making your carefully chosen shade look brash and brassy. Your personal color tint may start out looking beautifully balanced and in total harmony with your skin and eyes, but as you continue to shampoo, the color may begin to get brighter and brassier every time you wash it. That is a sure sign that your shampoo is to blame. When selecting a shampoo, look on the back of the container. Phrases like "recommended for tinted hair," "for delicate hair," or "will not strip color" are what you want to see. Also, as a general rule, the creamier the shampoo, the milder it will be on your hair. These gentle shampoos will get your hair just as clean as their stronger counterparts, but will not disturb the delicate balance of your color.

Further considerations in choosing the right shampoo for your color-treated hair include age, the length of your hair, and its natural texture:

- Young women in their teens and early twenties generally have active oil glands that affect the scalp and, in turn, their hair. They may need a shampoo with good cleansing ability, the type described as "for normal hair." Just make sure it has one of those key phrases that mean it will not strip color.
- Women with long hair may need a shampoo in the "normal" range, too, since their hair picks up more body oils than does short hair. Sometimes, though, long hair gets oily at the scalp but is dry on the ends. In this case, concentrate your shampooing at the scalp and rinse very thoroughly.

- If you have a perm or "relax" your hair in addition to coloring it, you'll need the most delicate shampoo. Your best bet is a shampoo that says "for dry or delicate hair" or "extra mild formula," and look for a nonstripping product.
- Wavy or naturally curly hair usually has good body, but what is surprising about this type of hair is that it tends to get dry very easily. Consequently, you need to conserve whatever moisture is present in your hair and should use the most delicate shampoo you can find. Look for a shampoo for permed hair, and you'll be on the right track.
- Soil shows up fastest on fine, thin hair, and if yours is a light color, it shows up that much more quickly. You will want to shampoo your hair often to keep it looking fresh, so your choice is in the "extra mild" and "delicate" category, too.

"Squeaky Clean Hair" and Other Myths

Squeaky-clean hair is a concept whose time has come—and gone. If your hair squeaks, after shampooing, you have stripped every bit of the natural oils off the surface and have *over*shampooed your hair. Also, you may be using a strong, old-fashioned shampoo that was originally designed to wash hair that was very soiled, and was intended to be used only once a week or every ten days. Also, for most modern women, shampooing *once,* then rinsing, is as much cleansing as hair needs. The old method of shampooing twice simply isn't necessary for hair that is cleansed every two or three days. There's a very logical conclusion to be drawn here: The more often you wash your hair, the less you have to scrub it and the less you have to strip the natural oils to keep it looking fresh and bouncy. Also, the more often you wash your hair, the milder the shampoo has to be, which results in less stress on your hair.

In the last few years the subject of pH balancing in shampoos has been discussed over and over. To me, this is another myth. Most shampoos on the market today are automatically formulated in the "mild" range, because the American woman washes her hair so often. Common sense would lead you to discontinue using a shampoo that was too strong or stripped your color. But making the pH factor in a shampoo the primary reason for buying it is really unnecessary. You have better methods of evaluating how a shampoo performs—by use-testing it!

Evaluating Your Shampoo

The ultimate test of a good shampoo is how your hair looks and feels after washing. If your hair takes a day or two to "calm down" after shampooing, that product may be too strong for your hair. If, on the other hand, your hair starts to look flat hours after it has been washed, you may need a shampoo that cleanses more effectively. There are many variables to consider in evaluating your shampoo. Do you exercise (and perspire) every other day? Is your hair oily by nature? Where do you live? If you live in San Francisco you'll need to shampoo less often than if you live in New York, where the air is much dirtier. Some trial and error is necessary, and you may add new variables every time you travel, change your hairstyle, stay on a diet for a period of time, take up a new sport, and so on. But after shampooing, your hair should look fresh, full, and shining. Don't settle for less.

Speaking of settling for less, don't succumb to a false sense of economy when it comes to buying a shampoo. You may have just bought one, tried it, and found your hair really isn't looking as good as it could. Because there's plenty of the shampoo left, however, you may decide to use it all up, even though your hair is looking less than wonderful. My advice is, if your shampoo isn't working on your hair, use the remainder on your lingerie and get something *great* for your hair! After all, your hair is one of the first things people will notice about you. So long as you use a mild shampoo, you can shampoo your hair every day, if you like, as we've discussed. Also, if you want to give your hair that extra touch of gloss, use *cool* water for your final rinse. It will "seal" the hair shaft and make your hair that much shinier.

The Need to Condition Regularly

There is no hair that does not look better when conditioned after every shampoo. The conditioner can be the simplest rinse-through variety, but it will give your hair increased luster and manageability.

When you shampoo your hair, you wash soil accumulation off the surface, or cuticle, of the hair strand. The cuticle, under a magnifying glass, has a structure of overlapping layers that look like fish scales. It is important that these layers lie flat and fit smoothly against one another if your hair is to reflect light well—and thus look shiny, lustrous, and healthy. Conditioners produce that smoothing effect, and that's why it is important to use them after shampooing, even if you *don't* color your hair.

If you've used any type of permanent color on your hair, using a conditioner becomes absolutely *mandatory.* Part of the permanent-coloring process (including highlights and frosting) involves a deliberate lifting of the cuticle, to enable the color or lightener to penetrate the hair shaft and reach the core of the hair. Thus, if you want your hair to reflect light brilliantly off a glossy surface, the cuticle will need smoothing down again. Conditioners do this perfectly and give the hair a smooth polish that enhances its natural shine.

Conditioners with Sunscreens

In addition to smoothing and shining up the hair, some conditioners contain a very important bonus: special sunscreening ingredients. In my opinion, this is one of the most important factors to consider in selecting a conditioner. There's no question that sun affects hair color drastically and will cause it to fade in direct relation to the amount of exposure. Visualize what happens to a living-room rug, one end of which is placed near a big window. The sun streaming through the window will bleach the colors of the carpet until that area no longer matches the rest of the rug. And that happens *indoors!* Exposing unprotected, color-treated hair to direct sunlight can cause similar results: The sun burns out the color and causes it to fade. Further, the sun creates a dry condition that makes color look totally flat. That is why using a conditioner with a sunscreen is a wonderful idea. Sunscreens conserve your color and prevent it from fading or going off. And even if you rinse most of the conditioning product off your hair after shampooing, the small amount that is absorbed by the hair protects your color and saves your hair from ultraviolet damage.

How to Comb Your Hair After Shampooing and Conditioning

You've been combing your hair all your life. What you may not know, however, is that there is a right and a wrong way of doing it. When hair is wet, it is at its lowest tensile strength because water adds extra weight to the hair and stretches it out to its maximum length. You've noticed this, I'm sure, when your hair is being trimmed: The stylist always allows for the fact that hair retracts and gets a fraction shorter as it dries. But while hair is wet and at its maximum extension, it is also at its most vulnerable to breakage.

If you stretch an elastic band as far as it will go, then try to stretch it more, it will snap. The same principle applies to wet hair. Stretch it any further, and it will break. That is why the first rule in handling wet hair is this: *Never* use a brush on wet hair. A brush pulls the hair past its maximum limit and can cause it to snap very easily. Instead of a brush, reach for a wide-toothed comb. Also, before actually combing the hair, towel dry to remove the extra water from the hair by squeezing it, not rubbing. Now here's how to comb wet hair the *right* way:

Using the wide-toothed comb, begin at the nape. Lift all the top hair with one hand and comb through the bottom-most section of wet hair with the other. Once you've combed through the hair at the nape, let some hair in the section above that drop, and work the comb through that section. Continue section by section, combing through each one separately, before dropping the one on top, until the comb slides easily through all the hair on the back of your head, up to and including the crown. Then repeat step by step on the left side and again on the right, combing through from *underneath* until all the hair is completely smooth. This method may be directly opposite to what you're used to doing: digging a comb in at the top of the crown and yanking it back down through the hair. Believe me, starting from the bottom and working *up* is a lot less painful and will do far less damage to your hair.

Too Little Conditioner

Just as young skin needs no more than a light moisturizing to restore its dewy balance, some hair needs no more than a light conditioning to keep it shining and reflecting light. But if you find your hair is beginning to look flyaway and fuzzy, it's time to consider a heavy-duty conditioner. This type of intensive conditioning for dry hair is the equivalent of a "cell renewal" cream for dry skin.

Frazzled-looking hair means the hair is thirsty and not getting enough moisture. Hair begins to look frizzy when it's colored or permed too frequently, or when color is put on top of a perm without conditioning enough in between. Electric appliances are a culprit here, too. The high wattage that allows you to speed up your blow drying can easily scorch the hair. The rule here is simple: the less, the better. Whenever possible, let color-treated hair dry naturally by itself; or at least let it dry partially on its own, then use a blow dryer to finish things off. When you do use a dryer, put it on one of the lesser cycles, under one thousand watts. And if you've been blowing your hair dry every day, try skipping a day in between. Hair is just as sensitive as your skin. Overusing a dryer is like giving your hair a sun- or windburn.

The treatment for dull, dry, fuzzy, flyaway hair is to condition, condition, condition. Regular treatments are a must. The type of product you should use for these heavy-duty treatments usually comes in a cream or oil form. You apply to the hair, leave on for at least fifteen minutes, then rinse thoroughly. Deep conditioning like this gives the hair a good, long drink of water and goes a long way toward preventing any further dehydration.

Most heavy-duty conditioners used regularly will give the hair new vitality, healthy-looking sheen, and accentuate its color highlights beautifully. Deep conditioning is the best way by far of treating hair that has suffered from heat, cold, hair-dryer abuse, or too much processing. Besides, regular conditioning treatments will not only restore the hair to every inch of its glorious potential, they will also *prevent* dryness and minimize further damage.

Too Much Conditioner

If you shampoo and condition only to find your hair feels as if you never washed it, you could be using the wrong conditioner. Conditioning should not make the hair feel heavy, limp, or too soft. On the contrary, it should make hair feel light, bouncy, and full of body. Some conditioners just make the hair easier to comb, but now that you know how to comb your wet hair properly, you don't need that type of product. Also, some ingredients are very difficult to rinse out of the hair—excess amounts of lanolin or jojoba oil, for example. If you find your hair feels weighted down after conditioning, start looking for a new, lighter product. There are hundreds of them out there that will do the job well.

If you highlight or frost your hair, you may be confused as to which type of conditioner (and shampoo, for that matter) to use. Essentially, you're dealing with two different types of hair at the same time, the color-treated strands and your own natural color. The lighter strands are more delicate, the natural hair stronger. What you should do is treat *all* your hair as if it were delicate, selecting the mildest shampoos and conditioners, so that you don't blanket the hair with too much of a good thing and leave it limp and flat. Using the lightest shampoo and conditioner will give your highlights the shine and intriguing light play they were designed to project.

Conditioners That Stay in Your Hair

In addition to conditioners you apply to your hair right after shampooing and those you use for heavy-duty treatments, there is another group of specialized conditioners designed to be left in the hair from shampoo to shampoo. Each of them has a particular purpose: to moisturize, to add body, to repair, to protect, to revitalize. None of them eliminates the need for regular deep treatments; they simply are a form of extra insurance that your hair will look its best at all times. Each is applied to towel-dried hair and on its container will tell you exactly what it will do for your hair.

For example, if you have fine, thin hair, a "body-building" conditioner adds extra volume and bulk to the hair, making it look much fuller and thus dramatizing the line of your hairstyle. A "moisturizing" conditioner is perfect for the woman whose hair has become dry, dull, or flyaway because of overexposure to heat, cold, or a dry climate. A small amount of this type of conditioner (usually in a very light creme form) does wonders in adding shine and healthy-looking luster to dried-out hair. Still another type of leave-in conditioner is designed to protect the hair from blow dryers, electric rollers, and curling wands. These "thermal" or heat-protective conditioners are very effective in creating a shield on the hair to help guard it against mechanical abuse. Protective conditioners of this type work beautifully and are a *must* if you use hair appliances on a regular basis.

One final example of a leave-in conditioner is the double-duty type that offers a repairing function at the same time that it *prevents* further damage. For the woman whose hair is dry and also in poor condition because of overcoloring or overperming, or from stress in the rest of her life, this type of product is a boon in regulating and conserving the moisture in the hair and scalp while it improves the elasticity of the hair. Words like "restores" or "revitalizes" signal that these products give your hair a livelier look and feel with more bounce and flexibility.

With all these products, the lighter the consistency, the better. After all, they're designed to be left in the hair, so you don't want to overload yourself with anything that dulls the hair's shine. One good way to test a leave-in conditioner is to apply a small dab or spritz on the back of your hand. If the product leaves an oily film on your skin, it will do the same thing on your hair. Look instead for a leave-in conditioner that almost disappears.

Another tip: Directions usually call for applying a "small" amount of the product to the hair. Believe them. Since leave-in conditioners stay in the hair until you shampoo the next time, don't drown your hair with pints of the product on the assumption that more is better. It isn't. *Less* is better, as long as you distribute the product evenly throughout the hair.

And one final point of information: Leave-in conditioners are *not* setting lotions. While these conditioners will make the hair more manageable, their main objective is to control and *improve the condition* of the hair, not to serve as a styling aid. This is a very important distinction. Don't expect extra hair-setting help from these conditioners. What they do best is to address particular hair problems. They'll add shine and lustrous gloss to hair while they heal a specific ill.

Salt Water, Chlorine, and Perspiration

For today's healthy, active woman, exercising and sports comprise a very important part of daily life. And there is no reason to limit any of these activities simply because you happen to color your hair. On the contrary, a well-toned body and a healthy glow to your complexion from exercising will complement hair that looks vibrant and healthy, too. Together they form the full picture of the energetic woman of the eighties. But since this is also the information decade, it helps to know what to avoid if you want to keep your beautiful healthy hair in its very best shape.

Salt water and chlorine are best avoided. However, if you don't want to stop submerging yourself in them, do avoid letting either one *dry* on your hair. Many of my clients enjoy swimming in the ocean; others swim laps in a pool for exercise. The real problems occur when salt and chlorine remain on the hair for periods of time, because they not only dry the hair, but also will distort the color and cause the hair to look dull, lifeless, and distressed.

The optimal ounce of prevention is to coat your hair lightly with a moisturizing cream or conditioner *before* stepping into the pool or ocean. This will make your hair look wet, but it's going to look a lot wetter before you're through, so what's the difference? Using conditioner as protection goes a long way toward avoiding any damage. However, if using conditioner in advance of your swim is not practical, the next best thing is to shampoo the salt or chlorine out of your hair *immediately* afterward. That will minimize the amount of time those strong agents are left in your hair causing trouble. If you don't want to precondition or can't shampoo right away, rinse your hair thoroughly with clear water as soon as you emerge from the ocean or pool. When you leave these strong elements in your hair you set off a chain reaction: Hair becomes faded and dry, so it has to be colored more frequently, and in turn conditioned more often, which means you're signing on for more hair care than you should need. Please follow this advice: Anytime your hair is exposed to salt or chlorine, at least *rinse* as soon as possible in order to keep your hair in good shape and your color glowing.

While salt and chlorine damage the hair, there is nothing quite as powerful as your own body's perspiration to create real havoc. Think what perspiration can do to a fine silk blouse. Perspiration penetrates fabric the same way it gets into the hair. Unless it's washed or rinsed out right away, you're going to have real problems. I've seen progressive photographs of color-treated hair that has faded because of salt or chlorine, but photographs showing the effect of perspiration on hair are more dramatic by far and exhibit the most profound deterioration of the hair's condition and color.

If you exercise enough to work up a sweat, be it outside or indoors, you should shampoo that perspiration off as quickly as possible to avoid doing serious damage to your color-treated hair. The faster you get it off the surface of the scalp and hair, the better. Everything that goes for salt and chlorine goes *double* for perspiration, because it poses a doubly serious threat to your hair's color and condition.

One more tip for athletes: Winding a scarf around your head during exercising will only heat up your scalp more and press the perspiration into your hair. If you're playing tennis or running, for example, I'd suggest you not wear a hat or scarf. Use a sweatband instead to hold hair off your face and absorb the perspiration. Depend on the sunscreen in your conditioner to protect your color. For the spectator watching an outdoor sporting event, a hat is fine. It will keep the sun off your face *and* your hair. Just make sure it's an open weave straw or mesh-type fabric so the breezes will circulate through your hair, keeping you cool and your hair "air-conditioned."

As you can see, I am absolutely passionate about keeping hair in its best possible condition. Hair color can be glorious, but if the hair that's wearing it looks like a piece of felt fabric, you've lost the entire point and fabulous impact color can have. There's nothing heroic, complicated, or even very difficult about taking care of color-treated hair. It's one of those simple follow-through routines of life, and one that makes all the difference in your good looks. If you've dieted and exercised properly, you have a slim, trim figure as your reward. All you have to do now is to practice a reasonable amount of maintenance. The hardest part is over. Coloring your hair is similar. Once you have radiant hair color, all you have to do is take proper care of it to continue to look your brightest, beautiful best.

17
Final Words
of Encouragement

My life's work is based on the conviction that hair color can do wonders for the way you look and feel about yourself. I see women transform their looks and their lives every day. Sometimes all a woman needs is a *small* change to give her an all-important boost in self-confidence. Sometimes her intuition tells her a *big* change is necessary. When she takes action on that hunch, the resulting improvement in her looks frequently triggers a series of changes that affect and improve the rest of her life, too.

I've been an eyewitness as well as a producer of those changes thousands of times, and the satisfaction of helping women achieve their greatest beauty potential is what keeps me so enthusiastic about what I do. And even though I may have worked with thousands of women so far, I look forward to each new day and meeting another new woman for the first time to see how I can help her begin to look her best. There's nothing as thrilling for me as to see a woman, who may have been unsure and tentative just a few hours earlier, walk out of my salon with a brand-new attitude toward herself and her life. I want you to feel that way, too. Confident, secure, indomitable, ready to take on *anything!*

Some of my clients started out with me during their student days when they simply wanted to have more fun with their hair. Over the years they've adapted their looks to suit different stages in their lives. They may have started out with temporary color or highlights, then progressed to permanent color, then to elegant frosting. Some look wonderful in a luminous, sparkling gray. Whatever your age or hair color right this minute, you can choose the method or shade that makes you feel best about yourself. Having read this book, you now know everything necessary to make a wonderful hair-color change for yourself. It's all there just waiting for you. *Do it!*

If you stop and think about it, everything about you has gotten better and better: your taste, your education, your ability to deal with people, your appreciation of art and music, the way you live. Your hair should reflect that improvement and be a part of it. Even if you don't consider your hair your very best feature, you can learn what it will do well and make that an asset. Fine straight hair shines like no other. Thick, curly hair holds the line of a good cut best. When you stop fighting your hair, go with what it does perfectly, then add the magical dimension of color, you'll be putting your hair into the right focus for the rest of your life and your own good looks. And when people look at you, they won't see pretty hair color, they'll see a pulled-together woman who cares for herself and who shines.

In many ways, having wonderful-looking hair symbolizes how you feel about yourself. When your hair is beautiful, you feel beautiful, you radiate confidence and send a signal to others that you care about yourself and about them, too. That's the feeling I want you to have.

You know that last look in the mirror you take on the way out the door? I want you to take that last quick look, pause for a second, and be able to say to yourself, "I look *terrific.*"

Index